Health and Hazard

Health and Hazard:
Spa Culture and the Social History of Medicine in the Nineteenth Century

By

Karl E. Wood

CAMBRIDGE SCHOLARS
PUBLISHING

Health and Hazard:
Spa Culture and the Social History of Medicine in the Nineteenth Century,
by Karl E. Wood

This book first published 2012

Cambridge Scholars Publishing

12 Back Chapman Street, Newcastle upon Tyne, NE6 2XX, UK

British Library Cataloguing in Publication Data
A catalogue record for this book is available from the British Library

ISBN (10): 1-4438-4099-8, ISBN (13): 978-1-4438-4099-6

TABLE OF CONTENTS

Acknowledgements vii

Chapter One 1
Introduction

Chapter Two 11
A Brief History of Spas to 1800

Chapter Three 25
The Romantic Spa 1800-1830

Chapter Four 61
The Price of Success 1830-1870

Chapter Five 95
Struggle for Survival: Curing Vice and Enlisting Science

Chapter Six 137
Conclusions

Chapter Seven 147
Epilogue

Appendix 155
Excerpt of *Hans-Jörgels Badereise*

Bibliography 165

Index 197

ACKNOWLEDGEMENTS

One often reads in dissertations that writing acknowledgements is the most satisfying part of the work. As I now write my own, I regard myself as fortunate to now be in the position to understand the truth of this statement. Expressing gratitude to those without whom this study never would have been possible provides a satisfaction greater than completing the work itself.

First and foremost, I would like to express my deep gratitude to my advisor, Richard S. Levy, whose intellectual astuteness, stimulating and constructive advice over the entire course of this work, as well as his humor and patient understanding for my unusual circumstances were invaluable. I cannot imagine having completed this work without his guidance. I also wish to thank my dissertation committee, Elspeth Carruthers, Astrida Tantillo, Kirk Hoppe and Katrin Schultheiss for their serious engagement with my work and their kind and valuable advice.

A number of scholars provided me with support throughout my research and writing. At the University of Illinois at Chicago, Marion Miller in her inimitable way helped give life to the project, and I wish to thank James Cracraft, Nicole Jordan, Michael Alexander, Leo Schelbert, and Christopher Boyer, each of whom assisted me in their individual ways to see my work to fruition. I wish to express my gratitude to those in Germany who helped guide me through the morass of possibilities for pursuing my research: Dieter Langewiesche and his seminar group at the University of Tübingen, as well as Wolfgang U. Eckart at the University of Heidelberg. I am also indebted to Aleksander Szwedek who lent me support and encouragement to bring the project to completion, and to David Blackbourn for his encouragement to investigate German spas.

Thanks also are due to Dagmara Kicherer of the Stadtarchiv Baden-Baden for her knowledgeable and friendly help and her faith in and enthusiasm for my project, to Herwig John and the staff of the Generallandesarchiv Karlsruhe as well as the staff at the Staatsbibliothek Preussischer Kulturbesitz zu Berlin for their kind assistance.

I wish also to express my gratitude for the financial support I was fortunate to enjoy: the German Academic Exchange Service for its research fellowship, the University of Illinois at Chicago for assistantships and fellowships throughout my graduate career, as well as Kazimierz Wielki University in Bydgoszcz.

A number of friends and colleagues stimulated me intellectually and gave me the help, support and comfort I needed so often during the process: Keith Green, James Kollenbroich, Nicole Butz, Sean Harris, Benn Williams, Linda van Puyenbroeck, Michael Johnson, and Maria Walat. My own parents and brothers, as well as my wife's parents were sources of strength without whom I could not have managed. My thanks also to Katarzyna Dudek for her strong moral support and her equally substantial desk on which the manuscript was written.

Finally, I most wish to thank my wife Edyta, whose keen eye for nonsense, inexhaustible patience, unconditional love, understanding, and sacrifice over many years were not only essential to my being able to complete this work, but in not entirely losing my wits in the process. I cannot thank her enough for this what I regard as our common success.

I am certain I have omitted thanks that are due to many others, a result no doubt of my own absent-mindedness at this stage. Despite all the assistance I have received, any and all errors and shortcomings of this work, of which there are many, are entirely my own.

CHAPTER ONE

INTRODUCTION

Warm waters bubbling forth from the earth, glamorous evening gowns and formal wear, orchestras and artists, casinos and promenades in the summer air –all these are images of the spa, that playground for fashionable nineteenth-century society. To this day, the thought of European health spas evokes something aristocratic, something sophisticated. However, these splendid places deserve more than nostalgia for a world past. They are worthy of serious historical study as important institutions that can tell us much of interest about European society in the past three centuries.

In its heyday in the nineteenth century, taking the waters was a popular and significant endeavor, showcasing much of what society had to offer. It was the place where social norms were set and broken, and rules of behavior were observed, enforced, and thwarted. Here rich and poor, aristocrats and commoners, maids and porters, bankers and bakers, lords, ladies, and ladies of the evening all had their prescribed roles in the drama set on the stage of the spa. In short, the spa represents a microcosm of the greater society that spawned it, although a unique one with its own peculiar culture.

This small world came to be dominated by the middle classes. In the eighteenth and early nineteenth century, royal courts made their summer residences at the spa, and the aristocracy ruled. Yet as the century progressed, the dominant social class became the bourgeoisie. The spa, like many other social, cultural, and political institutions became *bourgeois* or *bürgerlich*. As the middle classes came to populate the spas in increasing numbers and as their economic resources outstripped those of the aristocracy, their desires and priorities set the tone. For these resorts were commercial enterprises, often supported by the state, in intense competition with each other. In order to succeed, a spa had to offer what its paying customers wanted, or they would move on to a rival resort.

A wide range of activities was to be found at the spa: gambling, diplomacy, courtship, social interaction and representation were all important. Yet a core part of the experience, often neglected, is medicine.

For all the amusements that a spa offered, it was still at its core a place for medical treatment, where leisure and curing mixed in complementary fashion. Like leisure, curing was serious business.

The medicine of the fashionable spa world reveals a spectrum of competitive medical thought. Just as the nineteenth century was a formative time for middle-class identity, it was equally so for the modern science of medicine. As recent scholarship has shown,[1] this was the time of medicalization, during which the authority and position of scientific, positivistic academic medicine was established, while dissenting opinions were discredited and repressed. This result was not ensured, but was achieved by a complex interaction of the medical community and the state authorities and a shift in the attitudes of patients themselves. The rise to dominance of scientific medicine was not solely a top-down authoritarian procedure, but rather the product of an interplay of forces.

The spa offers a unique opportunity to the historian for the study of this process. Reflecting as it does middle class attitudes and the diversity of medical thought, the spa allows for examination of the relationship between medicine and society in this crucial formative period. With its middle class clientele seeking medical treatment of one form or another, and its practitioners representing competing schools of medical thought, the spa, although limited in space and scope, was diverse enough to yield illuminating examples of this dialogue between patient and practitioner, between state, medical establishment, and outsiders.

Several interpretive questions that bear upon this study have emerged from the debate over professionalization, medicalization, and patient autonomy. Alternatives to academic, allopathic medicine did gain popularity, yet establishment medicine ultimately came to dominate the world of medicine, both in practice and in attitudes. Was it the authoritarian-minded medical practitioner enforcing a monopoly over the

---

[1] See Michel Foucault, *The Birth of the Clinic; an Archaeology of Medical Perception* (New York: Pantheon Books, 1973) [1st American ed.]). Translated from the French (*Naissance de la clinique*) by A.M. Sheridan Smith. For the German context, see also Claudia Huerkamp, *Der Aufstieg der Ärzte im 19. Jahrhundert: vom gelehrten Stand zum professionellen Experten: das Beispiel Preussens* (Göttingen: Vandenhoeck & Ruprecht, 1985); Paul Weindling, *Health, Race and German Politics between National Unification and Nazism, 1870-1945* (Cambridge: Cambridge University Press, 1989); Jens Lachmund and Gunnar Stollberg, eds., *The Social Construction of Illness and Medical Knowledge in Past and Present* (Stuttgart: Franz Steiner, 1992). For an overview of the recent trends in the concept of medicalization, see also Robert A. Nye, "The Evolution of the Concept of Medicalization in the Late Twentieth Century," *Journal of History of the Behavioral Sciences* vol. 39, no. 2 (Spring, 2003), 115-129.

medical "market," acting in conjunction with the state, or a shift in mentalities and attitudes that precipitated this development? How did these two factors intersect and influence each other? Or on the other hand, was the development through which the traditional ideal of cultured generalists was splintered in favor of specialization more important? [2] Although at first it may seem far too limited and unique a world in which to examine these questions, in many ways, the very limitations of the spa offer a manageable and masterable space in which these and other questions can be studied.

It ought to be clear that much research remains to be done on this fascinating historical phenomenon. Because both medicine and society, particularly middle-class society, are well-represented in this milieu, it offers a forum quite suitable for an investigation of the intersections between the two, an investigation that has not yet been satisfactorily undertaken for the German context in particular.

German spa medicine was caught in the tension between academics and dissenters. This was particularly visible in the large, fashionable spas, or *Modebäder*, of which Baden-Baden was one of the most prominent. While certain smaller spas perhaps more clearly represented the alternative camp, most notably Wörishofen, home to the movement around Vincenz Priessnitz, a lay practitioner with no medical training, the *Modebäder* were host to the full range of conflicts outlined above. Spa administrations, usually subordinate to the local ministry of the interior and including academic physicians, were closely linked to the medical establishment of state and professional interest. At the same time, however, the field of balneology, as hydrotherapy came to be called after the 1850s, was struggling to maintain its position and reputation in the world of the medical academy and the medical community. Professionalization and medicalization are of particular interest in the *Modebäder*, as these lay on the fault line between alternative and academic, between the establishment and the resistance.

Over the course of the nineteenth century, the history of the spa can serve to outline developments in medicine which are hardly restricted to questions of practice and science, but which include questions of attitudes, both of practitioners and patients. As a prominent place both in the medical and social milieu, it can function as an historical laboratory for examining shifting mentalities. Medicine, tied as it is to modernity, is an important field of historical inquiry, and the spa represents an important

[2] Hans-Ulrich Wehler, *Deutsche Gesellschaftsgeschichte, Dritter Band: Von der "Deutschen Doppelrevolution bis zum Beginn des Ersten Weltkrieges, 1849-1914* (Munich: C.H. Beck, 1995), 735.

intersection of manifold social and scientific factors. Here, in the complex interaction of medicine and society, one can find explanations for how academic medicine came to dominance.

This question is worthy of study in any society, but it has a particular importance for German history. As the discussion of the professionalization of medicine in Germany suggests, German physicians acted in much closer cooperation with the state, and tended in time more toward conservative and indeed authoritarian practice. How the medical establishment fought alternative ways of thought, and tried to suppress them, can illuminate broader issues of society and mentality. The interaction of physicians and their patients, more generally, of medicine and society, can lead to a greater understanding of how authoritarian thought in general grew to be accepted by wide segments of the population. While this should not lead to a teleological search for Nazis lurking in nineteenth-century health spas, there is a link between the emergence of authoritarian thought in medicine and authoritarian political and social models that, in turn, contributed to the rise of National Socialism and may very well help account for the highly public role played by physicians during the Third Reich.

With this caveat in mind, the questions that this study will examine are ones of medicine and society in the spa. Possible answers to these questions can be sought in several areas of investigation, the first of which lies within the medical community. The manner in which professionalization manifested itself in the spa, and how professionalized, academic medicine asserted itself against practitioners outside the fold, is illustrative of the processes of exclusion of alternative ways of thought. Here the role of the physicians themselves, particularly within the state administrative structure, is a key area of examination.

The premise, however, that the acceptance of establishment medicine was also the product of patients' own developing attitudes, and not simply the result of the physicians' own professionalization projects, necessitates that the attitudes of the medical clientele be explored. This study will endeavor to use the *Modebäder* as a place to which patients were drawn, the sorts of decisions they made once there, and why they made them, all seen as reflective of their attitudes. In the spa as well, professionalized medicine grew more established as the century progressed; tracing the development of this trend, again in the spa milieu, can help illuminate the shift in particularly middle class attitudes toward medicine.

Beyond the enclosed spatial nature of the spa, other facets of the *Modebäder* make them well-suited to a study of the interaction of medicine and society. The *Modebäder* consisted of a mix of public and private institutions. Spa administrations, while nominally public institutions, often had owners of private clinics, hotel owners, and balneological physicians (*Bäderärzte*) as key members in the state administrative council. In this relatively well-defined arena, public and private medical interests are closely intertwined. The influence of private practitioners, of various kinds, on state policies can be directly observed in the spa world.

These spas were in keen competition with each other for visitors. Thus Baden-Baden competed with Bad Ems and Wiesbaden, as well as with resorts in France and Austria such as Vichy and Karlsbad. Competition for patients meant that these institutions can be studied as sensitive barometers of changes both in the medical field and in the desires and values of potential visitors.[3] The competition for patients and guests meant that the *Modebäder* constantly had to assess and re-tailor their services to the desires of potential guests, or see them take their business to another spa.

Spa administrations, as representatives of both the state interest and the local spa community interests, were charged with the task of ensuring that their resort remained competitive and would thrive. Throughout the century, one can observe the measures which the administrations took to further develop their facilities, to advertise, and to attract guests. While these measures included the building of theaters, parks, and other recreational facilities, much of the effort was concentrated specifically on ensuring that the medical bathing facilities within the town, both public and private, were up to the standards demanded by a discerning public and continually modernized. Advertising, targeted both at physicians who may refer patients and to the general public, focused primarily on the health benefits of a stay in the spa. The form that these efforts took, while on the one hand clearly reflecting the beliefs of spa physicians regarding what was the current state of the art, also must have reflected what they believed would be effective in attracting guests. Such advertising constitutes an important source for this study.

The *Modebäder* and their medical practitioners had to be responsive to the desires of their potential clients, but their advertisements and prescriptions no doubt also had an influence in shaping these desires as well. Neither the "top-down" model of medicalization nor the patient autonomy model can be taken in absolute form; rather, an interaction of factors determined the establishment of academic medicine. The study of medicine and society in the fashionable thermal health spas in Germany can yield some answers to the questions of medicalization and the ongoing

[3] Edward Shorter, "Private Clinics in Central Europe, 1850-1933," *Social History of Medicine* 3, no. 2, (1990), 159-195.

professionalization of medicine during the formative nineteenth century. In a spatially and temporally enclosed environment, one can trace the establishment of academic medicine over other schools of medical thought, both in concrete practice through state encouragement, and in the minds of middle class patients. By examining the responses of spa administrations and private practitioners, as well as the testimonies of spa patrons themselves, one can come to a better understanding of the complex, mutually formative interaction between popular attitudes and the professionalizing agenda of the medical establishment.

This study draws on a variety of source material, published primary and secondary sources, nineteenth century guidebooks, memoirs, and letters, as well as unpublished archival materials. Throughout the nineteenth-century, a large number of works were published on spas and spa medicine, growing in number as thermal spas grew more fashionable.[4] Spa descriptions and guidebooks of various kinds were prevalent throughout the century, extremely useful in registering changing perspectives, claims, and contentions. In general, these books must be viewed as a form of advertisement aimed at varying target audiences. Many were written by practicing balneologists or *Bäderärzte*, some were directed either at fellow physicians who might refer patients to the author's spa (and practice), others at the general public, and some at both. Fewer in number, but equally informative, are the guidebooks written by a layperson for the general public. What these guidebooks all have in common is a focus on the medical aspects of the spas. They attempt to portray their respective spas in the most attractive light possible, although not always uncritically, in order to attract visitors. Similar to these guidebooks are spa or balneological periodicals, which were edited by spa physicians, and directed at both the medical community and the general public.

Archival sources were available for this study in near-overwhelming variety and abundance. In order to render the project manageable, and to allow a greater depth of archival research, a single spa, Baden-Baden, one

[4] See for example, Konrad Anton Zwierlein, *Ueber die neuesten Badeanstalten in Deutschland* (Frankfurt: J.D. Simon, 1803); J. Franz Simon, *Die Heilquellen Europa's mit vorzüglicher Berücksichtigung ihrer chemischen Zusammensetzung* (Berlin: Albert Förstner, 1839); Friedrich Morin, *Die vorzüglichsten Bäder und Heilquellen Deutschlands und der Nachbarstaaten, deren ärztlichen Hülfen, Einrichtungen, Sehenswürdigkeiten, Vergnügungen und Umgebungen. Ein Rathgeber für Bade-Reisende* (Berlin: Nicolaische Verlagsbuchhandlung, 1867); K. Weller, *Taschenbuch für Badereisende. Jahrbuch der Bäder, Curorte, Heilanstalten 1873*. 5. verbesserte Auflage (Berlin: Denicke's Verlag, 1873).

of the most fashionable, and indeed, trend-setting thermal spas of the nineteenth century, has been employed as a case study. The archival materials for the *Modebad* Baden-Baden are shared between two archives: the *Stadtarchiv Baden-Baden* [City Archive of Baden-Baden] and the *Badisches Generallandesarchiv Karlsruhe* [Badenese General State Archive in Karlsruhe]. The materials available in these two archives include the records and documents of the spa administration, both in the city and at the state ministerial level, reaching as far back as the seventeenth century, and including for the nineteenth century thousands of pages of administrative correspondence, police and financial records, construction contracts, deliberations regarding advertising strategies, medical field officers' reports and letters of complaint from dissatisfied visitors. These records are indispensable for the study of the official level, and offer considerable insight into the interaction of private medical interest and state policy, of the development of the spas, and efforts to attract visitors in competition with other spas. Correspondence with other spas, in Germany and elsewhere, as well as minutes of spa administrative association meetings are also housed in these archives.

Spa patrons and patients also left behind documentation that the historian can access as primary source material. A range of published letters and memoirs offer insight into the quality of the spa experience.[5] This basis has been augmented and supplemented by nineteenth-century works of fiction set in the spa by a range of authors of varying degrees of fame.

Press accounts of spa life were common in nineteenth-century middle-class newspapers, particularly in the very popular *Morgenblatt für gebildete Stände* [Morning Press for the Educated Classes] published in Stuttgart and Tübingen from 1807-1867. These articles are useful, but must be read critically, for often a vested interest lay behind the publication. The publisher of the *Morgenblatt*, and the articles' likely author, was none other than the renowned publisher of Goethe and Schiller, Johann Friedrich Cotta, who also owned one of the most prominent bathing hotels in Baden-Baden. Other articles were written by

---

[5] Most letters and diaries written by ordinary persons remain unpublished; a large collection is available in the Schiller Archive of Manuscripts in Marbach, Germany. Unfortunately, these materials are difficult to access, not due to restrictions but rather owing to the manner in which they are catalogued. The collections of the Schiller Archive are indexed by author name only; a thematic catalog does not exist. As a regrettable result of time constraints, the archive could not be properly exploited for purposes of this study.

authors working on commission from the spa administrations, and, of course, were biased witnesses.

This work is structured in a chronological-thematic fashion, tracing the development of medicalization and the formation of middle-class society within the spa from 1815 to 1914. The main text is bracketed by a prologue covering the pre-1815 history of the spa and an epilogue that addresses the role of physicians and medical authority under Nazism. The introductory chapter discusses the history of the spa in the period prior to 1815. Although this period is not expressly part of the study, it provides the background out of which the nineteenth-century spa proceeded to develop. The following two chapters examine the beginnings of the modern spa through mid-century. Chapter Two investigates the birth of the modern spa, in the period from 1805 to 1830. In spa development, this was a period of considerable state support and guidance. For spa-visitors, this period witnessed the transition from the early period in which a spa visit was in first order a social and cultural experience, into a more medical experience. In medicine, which helped shape spa patrons' experiences, this was the period of Romantic medicine, based largely in Schelling's natural philosophy, which emphasized the mysterious healing properties of water. This foundation was essential: for the remainder of the century, spa physicians would attempt–with only partial success–to shake off the legacy of this formative period.

The third chapter focuses on the period of mid-century transformation, from 1830 to 1871. After 1830, the *Modebäder* were well-established: facilities were expanding and the number and diversity of visitors rising. Spa patrons increasingly sought curatives, and physicians of all kinds proliferated. This is the period of "*antimedizinische Flucht*"[6] [anti-medical flight], in which many looked toward natural remedies. This atmosphere was conducive to spa development, but also to the rise of lay healers claiming to make use of the waters. The period also witnessed the first attempts to establish spa medicine as a medical specialty–balneology.

The final period of the study is of the *Modebad* in Imperial Germany, to 1914. This is the period in which professionalization was well underway; it is also the period which saw the rise of wider popular movements critical of medicine. In this period the debates and tensions came to their greatest expression. Spa administrations attempted to establish the authority both of academic physicians against so-called

[6] For this term, as well as many thoughts regarding periodization and valuable insights into the tension between alternative and 'conventional' medicine, I am indebted to Professor Wolfgang U. Eckart of the University of Heidelberg. Personal correspondence to the author, October 29, 1999.

quacks (*Kurpfuscher*), or practitioners lacking full academic training. At the same time, these physicians were engaged in efforts to establish the scientific credentials of their field, balneology, as a truly scientific discipline, equal to all others of academic medicine. Spa visitors fell across the spectrum in their expectations. The number of visitors was higher than ever, as was the use of the balneological facilities. Many visitors sought what the "official" spa offered, yet others still came seeking alternatives, the therapies and treatments that the "quacks" offered. This last section examines these tensions between "establishment" medicine and "quacks," and attempts to answer the question of the establishment of medical authority within the context of health insurance schemes, which have been assigned a prominent place in the development of professional authority in Germany.

CHAPTER TWO

A BRIEF HISTORY OF SPAS TO 1800

Balnea, vina, Venus–baths, wine and Venus. These words inscribed on a tomb in Rome still speak their message across the centuries to the contemporary visitor.[1] The Romans' fondness for baths and concomitant sensual pleasures is legendary. But the marriage of the ancient elements of fire and water in thermal springs, issuing forth from the earth and filling the air with their pungent aroma in mineral baths was enjoyed not only by the Romans, but in cultures as diverse as those of Japan and Mesopotamia. These natural spring waters, predated and outlasted the Romans. The Empire fell, and in the provinces *thermae* fell into ruin. Many of these same springs which once had warmed the aching joints of legionnaires were used, centuries later, to treat Goethe and Bismarck. These ancient mineral springs became the elemental heart of the modern health spa.

A fundamental question in need of address at the outset of this study is what precisely *is* a spa? The term itself is ambiguous, referring generally in contemporary times to a host of trendy resorts offering a wide range of treatments designed to prevent illness or restore health once it is lost. The therapies offered are usually presented as alternative, that is to say an alternative to now conventional academic allopathic medicine, and may include massage, diet, herbal remedies, traditional Chinese medicine, Indian ayurvedic medicine, assorted meditation techniques as well as other essentially esoteric approaches to healing. Often located in remote areas in order to offer a pure environment, this modern incarnation of the spa is nonetheless a familiar sight to urban dwellers who can easily indulge themselves with a brief healthful sojourn in one of hundreds of "day spas" devoted to beauty, usually found in more affluent neighborhoods.

---

[1] *Corpus Inscriptionum Latinarum*, 6.15258. The full text as well as a translation of this passage of the inscription, *Balnea, vina, Venus corrumpunt corpora nostra, sed vitam faciunt b(alnea), v(ina), V(enus)* (Baths, wine, and sex ruin our bodies, but they are the essence of life –baths, wine, and sex) can be found also in Garrett G. Fagan, *Bathing in Public in the Roman World* (Ann Arbor: University of Michigan Press, 1999), 319, #261.

A cursory glance at the *Los Angeles Times*, for example, quickly reveals advertisements such as one for a "retreat into wellness with Dr. Andrew Weil at Sycamore Mineral Springs Resort"[2] in central California, where in five days participants can learn from the popular health guru how to "meet the demands of living without being overwhelmed." They can brace themselves for the struggle with the resort's health conscious nouvelle-cuisine restaurant and its therapeutic and leisure opportunities such as yoga and golf, all for the modest price of just under three thousand dollars, per person, double occupancy.

The contemporary spa, then, combines non-conventional medical approaches to health and wellness with leisure and relaxation in luxurious surroundings for those with the means. This fact raises the question, however, as to whether the spa, either in the contemporary world or historically, represents anything more than a coddling of the rich by means of an appealing exclusive vacation, with the fig leaf of (to some, dubious) medical treatment. The purpose of the present study is neither to evaluate the contemporary spa, nor to trace its development into the present, yet the example of Sycamore Springs shows striking similarities to spas of the past. Even in its modern incarnation, the spa has its origins in the nineteenth century, when travel as a sort of pilgrimage to spa towns in search not of salvation but of salubrity reached its apex of popularity, particularly in western Europe. To the historian versed in the history of the spa, the advertisements for Sycamore Mineral Springs, although expressed in a more modern cultural idiom, are highly reminiscent of nineteenth-century promotional literature for places such as Baden-Baden or Wiesbaden. The promise of health and leisure were then, as now, offered at a premium price to those with substantial means, while skeptics questioned the value of spa medicine.

What can be said about the spa from an historical perspective? The contemporary use of the word term only captures part of what can historically be understood as a spa. A place for healing or, depending on one's perspective, coddling the wealthy, omits an essential element of the historical spa which nevertheless is alluded to in the name of our California example: thermal mineral water. German terminology, despite the great importance of spa culture, is not altogether clear. A spa can be referred to in German as a *Kurort* [place of curing] or depending on the size of the locality, a *Kurstadt* [cure town]. Yet a *Kurort* may offer only fresh air–an "air cure," for pulmonary conditions, i.e., a *Luftkurort.* A

---

2 Advertisement in the *Los Angeles Times*, March 20, 2004, online edition, http://latimes.p2ionline.com/shoppingchannel/data/images/1109821.jpg.

proper spa may be referred to either as a *Badeort* or *Badestadt* [place of bathing or bath town], depending largely on the size of the municipality. Many of the more prominent spa towns contain either the word *Bad* [bath] in their names, such as Wiesbaden, or had the title conferred upon them by state authorities endorsing the salutary properties of the local springs such as Bad Ems or Bad Cannstatt near Stuttgart.[3] Yet bathing also includes seaside resorts, such as Norderney on the North Sea.[4] The precise definition of what constitutes a proper spa was and remains both slippery and contestable, but for the purpose of this study, a spa is understood as a resort town that offers therapy using thermal mineral water. Although other types of health resorts proliferated in the nineteenth century, mineral springs were the heart of the classic spa. Even as late as the 1970s, the Baltic seaside resort of Sopot (formerly Zoppot) felt mineral spring water important enough to go to the expense of drilling a deep well to offer the precious tonic from a fountain adjacent to the main medical clinic.[5]

Spas, then, require by definition mineral springs. These generally are found in mountainous areas and result from deep geological activity. One finds a belt of classic spas across the Pyrenees and in the Massif Central in France, in Southwestern Germany in the Black Forest and the Swabian Alb, in the Taunus mountains and the Rhineland, as well as in Austria, Bavaria, and topographically similar locales. It is in these areas that spas renowned for their waters are found, for example Vichy, Plombières, Evian, Bad Ems, Wiesbaden, Baden-Baden, and Bad Kissingen.

Much as contemporary spa promoters draw on the legacy of ancient health practices such as traditional Chinese medicine, to establish their credibility, nineteenth-century spa promoters were wont to make use of what they perceived, or wanted to have perceived by the public, as their own historical past. In German spas, this meant the legacy of the Roman past, especially after remains of Roman baths were unearthed and showcased early in the nineteenth century in many towns that then were popular spas, notably in Baden-Baden.

---

[3] The addition of the prefix *Bad* to a town name was a sought after pedigree and promotionally valuable, even as late as the 1960s, when Cannstatt became Bad Canstatt, signifying that a town was not simply a town, but a spa, or *Kurstadt*.

[4] For a superb and pioneering study of the growth of seaside resorts, see Alain Corbin, *The Lure of the Sea: The Discovery of the Seaside in the Western World, 1750-1840*. Jocelyn Phelps, transl. (Berkeley: University of California Press, 1994).

[5] Author's personal observations. The fountain, and the plaque commemorating its installation, are still found in the resort town in the heart of the resort area.

The Romans' fondness for baths and elaborate, some would say decadently ostentatious, facilities is widely known. Many of the greater Roman *thermae*, like the modern thermal spa, housed much more than simply baths; they were home to physicians, exercise and physical therapy, libraries, and even theaters. The *thermae* were open to all who could afford the admission fee, with the well-to-do bathing several times a day as a sign of their position and ability to devote themselves to leisure rather than cleanliness. This arrangement provided the opportunity for a wide range of social interaction, from the innocuous to the intimate.[6]

The Roman bath followed the advancing legions into the far reaches of the Empire. Across the Roman world, a city or even a private residence of substance had to include a proper bath, displaying luxury and the then high-technology of heat and large clear glass windows.[7] Bathing culture was adapted to particular conditions in the provinces; baths in the Gallican provinces could often have large heated basins in contrast to those in more temperate areas of the Empire.[8] In towns where thermal water was available, baths were constructed to take advantage of the springs. As a result, many modern spa towns can trace their origins back to the Romans. Baden-Baden was founded as the Roman Aquae in A.D. 70 (later renamed Aurelia Aquensis), Aachen was once Aquae Granis, and so on.

Beyond the construction of city and private baths, the Romans pioneered the concept of the resort spa. As the best-documented example, the town of Baiae was well established in antiquity as a locale that had all the requisite features to create an ideal playground for the public, including, importantly, hot mineral springs.[9] In ancient times such luxury offended moralists. To Cicero, Baiae was "a resort which encourages licentious conduct and wasteful lifestyle –idleness, debauchery, beach parties, boat parties, feasts, drinking."[10] Nor was Seneca convinced of the

[6] Vladímir Křížek, *Kulturgeschichte des Heilbades* (Stuttgart and Leipzig: W. Kohlhammer, 1990), p. 58.

[7] Klaus-Peter Goethert, "Badekultur, Badeorte, Bäderreise in den gallischen Provinzen," in Michael Matheus, ed., *Badeorte und Bäderreisen in Antike, Mittelalter und Neuzeit.* Mainzer Vorträge 5 (Stuttgart: Institut für Geschichtliche Landeskunde and der Universität Mainz/Fritz Steiner Verlag, 2001), 16-17.

[8] Gothert, "Badekultur, Badeorte, Bäderreise," 25 ff. See also Yaron Z. Eliav, "The Roman Bath as a Jewish Institution: Another Look at the Encounter between Judaism and the Greco-Roman Culture," *Journal for the Study of Judaism*, 31, no. 4 (November 2000): 416-454.

[9] Fikret K. Yegül, "The Thermo-Mineral Complex at Baiae and De Balneis Puteolanis," *Art Bulletin*, 78, no. 1 (March 1996): 137.

[10] Cicero, *Pro Caelio*, 15.35; also 16.38, 20.48-50, translated by and cited in Yegül, "The Thermo-Mineral Complex at Baiae," 137.

spa's appropriateness. After one brief stay, he described it as a "resort of vice (*deversorium vitiorum*)."[11] Baiae, for all its notoriety, was not the only resort of its kind in the Roman Empire; archeological evidence suggests that such places were also familiar in the provinces, including southwestern Germany. One such an establishment, near the Roman trade road from Trier to Mainz, had no other evident purpose other than providing a resort environment. The name of this resort has since been lost, but it is clear that it was associated with the cult of Asclepios, or in the Romano-Celtic region, Apollo Grannus,[12] and resembled the Hellenistic *Asclepieion*, dedicated in other regions of the Empire to Asclepios, the Greek god of healing, whose staff entwined with snakes still serves as the symbol of modern medicine.[13] The *Asclepieion* had many features that are later found in the modern thermal spa: varied medicinal use of mineral waters for a range of maladies, facilities for dining and rest, and a theater as well as other amusements. All of these, as with the modern spa, were regarded as important elements of the whole therapeutic experience.[14]

As the Roman Empire crumbled, however, so too did the culture of the baths. The famous baths of Rome itself fell into disuse; Roman towns east of the Rhine were often abandoned or destroyed and with them, their baths. Aurelia Aquensis disappeared entirely from the historical record at the time of the Germanic invasions in A.D. 260, until it reappeared as Baden in documents of the tenth century.[15] Some Roman baths such as Baiae may have continued to be used well into the Middle Ages,[16] but it is all but certain that in areas conquered by Germanic tribes, the waters and spas were abandoned. Although this legacy later provided inspiration for nineteenth-century imaginations, the modern Central European spa cannot claim an unbroken descent from the Roman *thermae*.

By the twelfth century, however, evidence in the form of manuscripts and claims, both authentic and forged, to mineral springs, testifies to a renewed interest in their use. Sources regarding the Early Middle Ages are

---

[11] Seneca, "On Baiae and Morals," Letter 52, translated by and cited in Yegül, "The Thermo-Mineral Complex at Baiae," 137.

[12] Goethert, "Badekultur, Badeorte, Bäderreise," 28.

[13] See Michael T. Compton, "The Association of Hygieia with Asklepios in Graeco-Roman Asklepieion Medicine" *Journal of the History of Medicine and Allied Sciences* 57, no 3 (2002): 312-329.

[14] Křížek, *Geschichte des Heilbades*, 35-36.

[15] Rolf Gustav Haebler, *Geschcihte der Stadt und des Kurortes Baden-Baden*, Second Edition (Baden-Baden: Verlag Dr. Willy Schmidt, 1969), 1: 40.

[16] Yegül, "The Thermo-Mineral Complex at Baiae," 138.

limited, but they do suggest that local watering places were indeed frequented. The statutes of the Zurich cathedral from 1376 promise the canons there biannual paid leaves for a trip to nearby Baden im Aargau, which was then a popular destination. Similarly, in the fifteenth century, high officials of the city of Nuremberg were entitled to a leave to visit a thermal bath.[17]

The fifteenth century witnessed a rapid expansion of thermal bathing establishments, either at so-called "wild baths" [*Wildbäder*] which offered open thermal waters in a provocatively dangerous environment of untamed nature, or more securely within walled towns which provided an element of security to vulnerable bathers.[18] Travel reports and letters from this period document a lively spa culture in popular destinations such as Baden im Aargau, Baden-Baden, and Wiesbaden. Bathers included the noble and burghers alike. In a relatively well-known account from 1416, an Italian Renaissance traveler, Poggio Bracciolini renders a vivid portrait of a sojourn in Baden im Aargau, detailing the socially elite visitors' frivolity and indulgence in lascivious pleasures. This literary evidence largely squares with artwork surviving from the period, which commonly portrays nude bathers of both sexes sharing not only a common basin, but uninhibited sexual expression as well.[19] Yet Poggio's account was likely an exaggeration, written to entertain a friend and obliquely to criticize Italian mores using the "noble savages" north of the Alps as a foil.[20] When balanced with other historical documents, such as Paracelsus' descriptions of thermal waters or a travel account by Hans von Waltheym, a German salt merchant, a more complex picture emerges. Certainly amusement and licentiousness were part of the experience, but this was more a diversion from the primary purpose of such a trip, which was curative.

Yet in spite of the healthful purpose of taking the waters, an image of libidinous carousing emerged that incensed moral opponents who lambasted the decadence and frivolity of the baths. Thus Cicero's contempt reappeared as a veritable leitmotif in perceptions of the spa and spa culture. On the one hand, the waters themselves were seen as a

---

[17] Birgit Studt, "Die Badenfahrt. Ein Neues Muster der Badepraxis und Badegeselligkeit," in: Michael Matheus, ed., *Badeorte und Bäderreisen in Antike, Mittelalter und Neuzeit*, 35.

[18] Mathias Bitz, *Badewesen in Südwestdeutschland 1550 bis 1840* (Idstein: Schulz-Kirchner Verlag, 1989), 41.

[19] See for example the color plates in Gernot von Hahn and Hans-Kaspar von Schönfels, *Wunderbares Wasser. Von der heilsamen Kraft der Brunnen und Bäder* (Aarau, Stuttgart: AT Verlag, 1980), 68-72.

[20] Studt, "Die Badenfahrt," 43.

positive thing, but nudity and relatively loose atmosphere, some morally minded critics felt, undermined both proper mores and the curative effects of the waters. Such assaults had some concrete results: by the sixteenth century, many monastic orders, giving expression to the moralizing impulse which baths provoked, prohibited their members from undertaking a *Badenfahrt*, and if one was regarded as absolutely necessary for health reasons, strict moral guidelines were to be observed.[21] By the 1700s, communal bathing tubs, which had been the custom in the preceding centuries, virtually disappeared; bathing itself had become either a private matter in individual cabinets, or had fallen completely into disfavor. Fueled by the moralists' denunciations, an increased sense of shame regarding nudity and the very real spread of syphilis which had become endemic to urban bathhouses, the changing fashions of behavior were such that the middle and upper strata of society had nearly entirely eschewed daily bathing by the second half of the seventeenth century.[22]

Moralizing voices that condemned pleasure, however, were not the only voices to be raised. Aside from the tendency to condemn anything in the spa not strictly connected with curing, a contrary view sought to justify spa amusements as an integral and healthful part of the healing process. Exemplary for this new direction was Heinrich Bebel, an academic in Tübingen. For Bebel, amusement and curative bathing were intricately linked, working together in harmony. Both were necessary in order to achieve a successful cure. This is one of the earliest expressions of a theme that became central to spa culture: leisure at the spa was not supplementary to medicine, but in fact as much part of a therapeutic regimen as mineral waters, laxatives, and bloodletting.[23]

The net effect of these trends was a changed spa, although not necessarily changed in the ways that moralists would have envisioned. In place of extended baths in open basins, the drinking cure increasingly came into vogue–quite satisfactory, no doubt, to those offended by communal baths. But in place of the socializing that had previously taken place in the tubs, a new sociability came to the fore in the spa of the seventeenth century.

Until the 1600s, the spa was a gathering place for local elites and the occasional traveler. Baden-Baden hosted mainly visitors from nearby Strassburg, Baden im Aargau from nearby Zurich, and so on. The social composition of the curing public tended to represent a mix of wealthy city-

[21] Studt, "Die Badenfahrt," 48.

[22] Bitz, *Badewesen in Südwestdeutschland*, 137. See also Sigfried Gideon, *Geschichte des Bades*, (Hamburg: Europäische Verlagsanstalt, 1988), 32-34.

[23] Studt, "Die Badenfahrt," 48.

dwelling merchants, clergymen and the local nobility, mingling not infrequently with the poor sent for a cure on public alms. The communal basins of the sixteenth century hosted rich and poor alike, even the occasional horse could be found taking the same waters. By the dawn of the eighteenth century, however, the spa began to fill another role, functioning as a sort of summer court with a corresponding growth of exclusivity.

Spa towns enacted legislation aimed at the maintenance of order within the spa district. A clear purpose, of course, was to ensure the safety of wealthy patrons, who often became victims of crime. An indication of the variety of indignities they were subject to may be seen in the actions taken by Count Georg of Hessen-Darmstadt, who in 1630 designated a special "peace zone" in the spa town of Langenschwalbach, where "the carrying of weapons, shoving, striking, or even improper touching of persons" was punishable by having the offender's hand chopped off. Langenschwalbach, however, lacked city walls, and despite additional night watchmen, the measures could only be partially successful.[24] In more settled spa towns, such as Wiesbaden, the walls and city gates provided a minimal element of security, in that dubious characters could more easily be kept out of the town altogether.

Exclusion of "unsuitable" elements from the curing district of the eighteenth-century spa was important not just for the comfort and safety of the more "respectable" visitors, but rather also because the spa itself had been discovered by the state. In previous centuries, spa towns had attracted visitors by virtue of their waters and their guesthouses; by 1700 a new model of princely or state sponsorship was emerging. The most successful spas of the eighteenth century were those, which enjoyed state support. Spas were attractive, especially to small states, because they helped fill empty coffers. With this hope in mind, for example, Prince Georg August of Nassau launched a program of modernization and promotion in Wiesbaden in 1690. His successors continued his work, improving the gardens, attracting French and Savoy merchants and engaging traveling theatre companies, so that by 1765, Wiesbaden could be regarded as an exemplary case of successful spa promotion by state authorities.[25]

The desire among mercantilist-minded princelings to attract revenues to their territories was but one motive for spa promotion in the eighteenth

[24] Martina Bleymehl-Eiler, "Das Paradies der Kurgäste' - Die Bäder Wiesbaden, Langenschwalbach und Schlangenbad im 17. und 18. Jahrhundert." in: Michael Matheus, ed., *Badeorte und Bäderreisen in Antike, Mittelalter und Neuzeit,* 69. This and all subsequent translations, unless otherwise noted, are my own [kw].
[25] Bleymehl-Eiler, "Das Paradies der Kurgäste," 60-63.

century. Of greater importance was a desire to create a showcase town. Much as Louis XIV built Versailles as a representation of the splendor of his monarchy, some lesser German princes turned to spa construction to represent their reign and advertise their glory. So, the small spa of Bad Brückenau near Fulda visibly and tangibly reflected the absolutist aspirations of the ruler in its high baroque palace and curing facilities.[26] This impulse gave rise to its own architectural style, with the emphatically palatial structures supplanting the sparely functional.[27] Key features of the spa, from the monumental drinking hall with relaxation spaces to the elaborately landscaped gardens for leisurely strolls, became typical fixtures of the aristocratic spa in the eighteenth century.

Aristocratic in its demeanor and accoutrements, the spa began attracting increasing numbers of middle-class patrons during the course of the eighteenth century. One of the key factors in this development was the conscious promotion of medicine and curing. Awareness of illness as something that could be ameliorated by the healing waters of the spa grew among the educated public at this time, drawing greater numbers of rich and poor, the infirm and the bored who hoped to recoup their health at resorts featuring natural springs.[28] Sensing this tendency, and eager to attract guests who would enhance the revenues of the prince-sponsor of the spa, many commissioned medical treatises as a form of promotional literature. Indicative of this trend was Baron Konstantin of Hesse who was interested in his spa Langenschwalbach as a financially profitable enterprise, sponsored "studies" of the medicinal benefits of the spring waters in the 1740s.[29] While luxury and high society might appeal to the aristocracy, the findings of science were more likely to attract the bourgeois reading public. Spa promoters, especially physicians, tried to cast as wide a web as possible, making near panacea claims for the healing waters in order to attract the largest number of ill and convalescents as possible.[30]

[26] Burkhard Fuhs, *Mondäne Orte einer Vornehmen Gesellschaft. Kultur und Geschichte der Kurstädte 1700-1900.* Historische Texte und Studien, vol. 13 (Hildesheim, Zürich, New York: Olms Verlag, 1992), 27.
[27] Fuhs, *Mondäne Orte einer Vornehmen Gesellschaft*, 38-39.
[28] Barbara M. Benedict, "Consumptive Communities: Commodifying Nature in Spa Society." *The Eighteenth Century* 36, no. 3 (1995): 203. See also Reinhard Kuhnert, *Urbanität auf dem Lande. Badereisen nach Pyrmont im 18. Jahrhundert* (Göttingen: Vandenhoeck & Ruprecht, 1984), 59-73.
[29] Bleymehl-Eiler, "Das Paradies der Kurgäste," 70.
[30] Kuhnert, *Urbanität auf dem Lande*, 60.

Medical treatment at spas no doubt drew a significant number of visitors, yet the intimate quarters of a small spa town also offered another attraction, perhaps equally as important, sociable communication and interaction. A summer sojourn in a spa allowed visitors to amuse themselves and, at the same time, to make new acquaintances or to renew old ones.[31] This supplemented, rather than replaced, the era's vibrant literary culture of letter writing to allow interregional contact between individuals. The spa, then, formed a sort of community, offering the leisure and curative opportunities of a retreat from urban life, while retaining the sophisticated character of an urban center, from which most of the middle-class guests came. As one contemporary observer and visitor to Pyrmont observed:

> One is far from the court and the city, and grand society, in peaceful environs; but the court, the city, and grand society are there, too; one is in the country, surrounded by all the trappings of the city.[32]

The outward symbols of princely and aristocratic power also lured middle-class visitors with social ambitions. The splendid thermal towns served as the summer courts of many princes, and as such, drew those seeking to integrate or ingratiate themselves with the centers of power. These spas, while exclusive to the extent that the poor and unsightly were marginalized or excluded, remained open to the "better" orders of society. Clearly, distinctions were made, not all were equal in the spa, but the relative openness of this courtly institution provided a unique environment in which the rising middle classes could participate, and thus reduce the tensions between prince, nobility and *Bürgertum.*[33] Because the German lands lacked a great national capital, like Paris or London, the German spa was particularly important as the provider of an urbane venue for social interaction.[34]

The spa, then, was only one stage for a development of much larger significance. The eighteenth century saw the beginnings of the entrance into elite society by the educated middle class. Certainly, this process had begun earlier, in the seventeenth or even sixteenth century with large merchant families operating in cities and towns, but it was in the

---

[31] Kuhnert, *Urbanität auf dem Lande*, 77.

[32] Jens Baggesen, *Humoristische Reisen durch Dänemark, Deutschland und die Schweiz*. 4: 163 (Mainz, 1801), cited in Kuhnert, *Urbanität auf dem Lande*, 93.

[33] Fuhs, *Mondäne Orte*, 49.

[34] Reinhold Kuhnert, "Badereisen im 18. Jahrhundert–Sozialleben zur Zeit der Aufklärung," *Journal für Geschichte*, no. 1 (1987): 17.

eighteenth that the emergence of an educated elite, influential in areas of court, military, local politics, and state administration, as well as finances and trade, a new *Bürgertum*, conscious of itself and possessing a confident, trans-regional identity, began to coalesce.[35] These changes, much further advanced elsewhere, were slow to develop in German-speaking Europe, and the middle classes there were still far from imposing.[36] But its rise to power and significance in the nineteenth century began with its gradual penetration into elite circles. The spa offered this opportunity without much in the way of fanfare.[37]

The spa in the later eighteenth century was well-suited to play an important role in this process. Its relatively relaxed and inclusive atmosphere contributed to the erosion of the barriers between the *Stände*, within the bourgeois and to an extent, between bourgeois and noble, forming the beginning of a hybrid status, lying somewhere between an aristocratic and a bourgeois society.[38] Here the bourgeois could assert themselves, modestly, to be sure, always showing the proper respect in the presence of nobles. Such contact took many forms, for example, a bourgeois extending breakfast invitations to nobles, or shared participation in excursions or balls which in the past had been the exclusive realm of the aristocracy, or a shared taking of the waters in the *Trinkhalle*, where mineral water for therapeutic drinking was dispensed.[39]

This opportunity for shared experiences between bourgeois and noble was discernible enough to contemporaries to call forth a new term, "spa

---

[35] Lothar Gall, *Von der ständischen zur bürgerlichen Gesellschaft,* (Munich: Oldenbourg, 1993), 13-14.

[36] David Blackbourn, "The German Bourgeoisie: An Introduction," in: David Blackbourn and Richard J. Evans, eds. *The German Bourgeoisie. Essays on the Social History of the German Middle Class from the Late Eighteenth Century to the Early Twentieth Century* (London and New York: Routledge, 1991), 4.

[37] The emergence of the bourgeoisie in the late eighteenth and nineteenth centuries has been the subject of a considerable body of scholarly research. In addition to Gall, *Von der ständischen zur bürgerlichen Gesellschaft* and Blackbourn and Evans, *The German Bourgeoisie* (cited above), see for example, Werner Konze and Jürgen Kocka, et al. eds., *Bildungbürgertum im 19. Jahrhundert.* 4 volumes (Stuttgart: Klett-Cotta, 1985-92); Lothar Gall, *Bürgertum in Deutschland* (Berlin: Siedler, 1989); Lothar Gall, ed., *Stadt und Bürgertum im 19. Jahrhundert* (Munich: Oldenbourg, 1990); see also the two current works of general synthesis by Hans-Ulrich Wehler, *Deutsche Gesellschaftsgeschichte*, 5 volumes (Munich: C.H. Beck, 1996-2003), and Thomas Nipperdey, *Deutsche Geschichte* 3 volumes, Brochierte Sonderausgabe (Munich: C.H. Beck, 1998).

[38] Fuhs, *Mondäne Orte*, 47.

[39] Kuhnert, "Badereisen im 18. Jahrhundert," 21.

freedom" (*Badefreiheit*). As one observer wrote, "…interaction is easy and unrestrained … Without reservation one can address anyone to whom one had been introduced, or even introduces oneself; one can approach any circle one desires to take part in the conversation."[40] This description of easygoing social freedom ought not be taken absolutely literally; it may have reflected wish as much or more than reality. The barriers between the *Stände* remained intact, and outside the spa, often impermeable. Inside the spa, however, the social boundaries seem to have become somewhat easier to cross. "Spa freedom," while not to be confused with equality, signified for the elite bourgeois guest a heady departure from the conventional deference due the aristocracy, and one can imagine, that even this appearance of complete freedom must have had an exhilarating effect. No doubt, it accounts for some of the spa's growing appeal for middle-class patrons.

The twilight of the eighteenth century brought with it significant disruption of the world of the aristocratic spa in the wake of the French Revolution and Napoleonic warfare. In its place, a new incarnation of the spa, oriented toward a moneyed bourgeoisie, gradually replaced the courtly predecessor. This new spa that came fully into its own in the early nineteenth century enjoyed state sponsorship, but it also developed into an unabashedly commercial enterprise, subject to market forces and dependent on pleasing the consumer. The aristocratic spas of the eighteenth century, few in number and fairly limited in size, did not altogether disappear but nor did they thrive in the new age. Pyrmont lingered on in obscurity while other spas emerged as the new haunts of *bon ton* society. Those that could not adapt to the new demands of a changing clientele or compete for their business were marginalized or disappeared entirely.[41]

The new spa that arose in the era of Romanticism was to attempt to invoke the legacy of the past as part of their appeal. The lack of direct continuity from Rome, certainly did not discourage nineteenth-century spa promoters from exploiting any shred of Roman legacy they could find. As shall be discussed in Chapter Three, museums exhibiting Roman artifacts were displayed prominently in Baden-Baden after 1804, elaborate steam bath facilities were constructed clearly based on Roman models, and guidebooks for visitors consistently evoked the Roman past of spa towns. Local histories written in the nineteenth century, too, made much of this

---

[40] H.M. Marcard, *Beschreibung von Pyrmont 1-2 und Ergänzungsband mit Kupferstichen* (Leipzig, 1784/85), cited in Kuhnert, "Badereisen im 18. Jahrhundert," 18.

[41] Fuhs, *Mondäne Orte*, 42.

legacy, consciously trying to establish a link of continuity with Rome. Writers made much of the visit of the Roman emperor Caracalla, claiming boldly (and without evidence) that his visit to Aurelia Aquensis inspired the construction of his monumental baths in Rome. A later author and spa physician dismissed such grandiose claims, but suggested a (highly dubious) continuity of development from Hadrian to the Baden-Baden of the nineteenth century. Although such claims were based on manuscripts later exposed as forgeries,[42] and the claims of a direct line of descent were evidently bogus, the perception of classical heritage was one part of a promotional strategy that propelled the spa to its zenith of popularity in the nineteenth century.

[42] Franz Heiligenthal, *Geschichte der Stadt Baden und Ihrer Bäder* (Karlsruhe: Braun'sche Hofbuchdruckerei, 1879), 6. See also Haebler, *Geschichte der Stadt und des Kurortes Baden-Baden*, 1: 36-38.

CHAPTER THREE

THE ROMANTIC SPA 1800-1830

"Taking the waters" took a quantum leap in popularity in the first decades of the nineteenth century, prompting a period of expansion for thermal health spas in German lands. An ever larger number of visitors frequented these tranquil refuges from the tumult of an eventful era. The number of guests in Baden-Baden, the focus of this study, rose from an average of 320 visitors annually in the 1790s to over one thousand annually in the first decade of the nineteenth century, 3,398 in the 1810s, and 7,398 in the 1820s. [1] A similar trend was discernable for Wiesbaden, Baden-Baden's main rival, which saw its number of guests nearly double between 1800 and 1820.[2] People began to flock to spas, and formerly little known spas became fixtures on the in vogue circuit, their reputation for sophistication spreading far and wide. An early witness to these developments, the spa physician, K.A. Zwierlein, wondered aloud about this change in his world and broached many of the vexed questions that have puzzled interpreters of the phenomenon ever since: "Have people become more convinced of the usefulness of the baths for their health? Or is it a now fashionable luxury? Or perhaps charlatan deception?" He concluded that each of these factors was instrumental in the undeniable

---

[1] Statistics from the Baden-Baden Guest Registry (*Fremdenliste*), 1790-1800 cited in Johann Loeser, *Geschichte der Stadt Baden* (Baden-Baden: Sommermeyer, 1891), p. 281 and "Fremdenliste der Stadt Baden während des 19. Jahrhunderts,", p. 429. Averages are given because annual figures could vary considerably, given the turbulence of the Napoleonic era. In 1781, for example, 662 guests visited Baden-Baden, while in 1796, the figure was a meager 52.

[2] Mathias Bitz, *Badewesen in Südwestdeutschland 1550 bis 1840. Zum Wandel von Gesellschaft und Architektur* (Idstein: Schultz-Kirchner Verlag, 1989), 312. Exact figures are not given, but rather represented in a graph showing the trends for Baden-Baden and Wiesbaden.

popularity of bathing establishments generally, the luxurious thermal spas being the most fashionable and desirable of these.[3]

What was it that guests sought in these places? Fashion, leisure, and social interaction all had a role to play, but spas—it should not be overlooked—were also places of curing, *Kurorte*. On this much bathers and physicians could agree: in moderation, leisure *was* part of a therapeutic regimen. The medicinal use of the waters, the first of Zwierlein's points, was integrated together with amusement and social rituals to construct the entire experience. Curing and pleasure were joined in one place dedicated, in principle, to the pursuit of health through the purportedly powerful salutary properties of the waters.

This integration of leisure and healing was not new, nor was the place of physicians in the spa. In the early modern period, when the "drinking cure" replaced extended communal baths as the mode of choice for taking the waters, physicians made their presence felt in spring towns. By the 1600s, they were frequently established as practitioners, consulted both by visitors and by state authorities regarding the most effective use of mineral waters. This put them in a position in which they could exert their influence, and from the eighteenth century onward, physicians had a considerable role in shaping the spa experience.[4]

Along with patrons and physicians, the state was another keenly interested party in the developmental expansion of spas. Governmental authorities, seeing to the prestige of the state, supported their growth with financial and administrative means. As a result, little-known towns in German lands grew into cosmopolitan spas, with facilities for both medicine and entertainment being constructed simultaneously. Spa development reflected the vested interest of all the key players: a medical establishment of mounting influence, a state anxious to serve its own interests, and middle-class visitors eager for what they thought the spa could give them.

In this environment where medicine and leisure blended together, the historian can observe the complex of forces that defined the spa in the first decades of the nineteenth century. The Romantic period was formative for the modern health spa. It witnessed the construction and promotion of new establishments, both private and public, that were tailored to meet the manifold expectations of their mostly bourgeois guests. How these needs were defined and then accommodated, and how they interacted with the

[3] Konrad Anton Zwierlein, *Ueber die neuesten Badeanstalten in Deutschland.* (Frankfurt: J.D. Simon, 1803), iii–iv.
[4] Bitz, *Badewesen in Südwestdeutschland*, 82.

aspirations of academically trained physicians struggling for status and recognition, form the central questions for this chapter.

Baden-Baden, as a spa that rose quickly from obscurity to prominence, provides an example well-suited to this investigation. The waters had been used for medicinal purposes by the Romans in the settlement of Aurelia Aquensis as early as A.D. 70. But the town disappeared from the historical record for several centuries, and appears to have been abandoned, reemerging only in the Middle Ages, this time as a place of curing for local inhabitants. In the late medieval period, referred to by chroniclers as a "golden age," Baden-Baden was a princely residence that hosted visits by the Holy Roman Emperor and other lofty personages. This glory ended in 1689, when burnt to the ground by French troops, the town was reduced to a torpid ruin.[5] Through most of the eighteenth century, Baden-Baden remained a sleepy provincial town. Only with the dawn of the nineteenth century did this change.

In 1805, Baden-Baden saw just over 1,200 visitors a year, mostly from the surrounding area, including the poor and indigent.[6] Guest registries (*Kurlisten*–discussed in greater detail below) from 1805, for instance, reveal a handful of nobles and predominantly educated middle-class visitors, such as professors traveling with students, pastors, and businessmen traveling with or without their wives.[7] Two decades later the spa was well-established on the international scene, hosting 8,364 guests consisting mostly of "excellent men … from the most preferable parts of the middle class" as well as noble visitors from "distinguished families" and respectable visitors from abroad, especially England and France, making 1826 the best yet, both in the number and the "quality" of guests.[8] From a position of bucolic obscurity at the beginning of the century, Baden-Baden by 1830 had arrived on the international circuit of taking the waters.

---

[5] Rolf Gustav Haebler, *Geschichte der Stadt und des Kurortes Baden-Baden*, vol. 1, (Baden-Baden: Verlag Dr. Willy Schmidt, 1969), chapters 4 and 5.

[6] Generallandesarchiv Karlsruhe Signatur 195/294 (Hereafter referred to in short format as GLAKa 195/294), "Nummarischer Extract aus den Scheinen der Badgastwirthe wegen allen von Anfang der diesjährigen Badkurzeit bis zum Ende derselben, nähmlich von Georgi bis Michaelj, 1805, Gubrauchung der Badkur in Baden sich eingefundenen Fremden," October 7, 1805.

[7] GLAKa 195/1062, "Gedruckte und handschriftliche Verzeichnisse der Kurgäste in Baden-Baden. 1807." Guest registries from 1807 which listed visitors' names and professions. For a detailed analysis of the social composition of these lists in Bad Ems, see Hermann Sommer, *Zur Kur nach Ems, ein Beitrag zur Geschichte der Badereise von 1830 bis 1914* (Stuttgart: Steiner, 1999).

[8] GLAKa 195/988,"Generalbericht über den hiesigen Kurort" for the season 1826.

This had clearly been the intent of the resort-town's sponsor, the government of Margrave Karl Friedrich of Baden, that undertook measures to improve the bathing and entertainment facilities in Baden-Baden beginning in the late eighteenth century. These were pursued in earnest after 1806, when Karl Friedrich, newly elevated to the Grand Duke of Baden, established his summer residence in Baden-Baden. It was the tangible and concerted efforts of the state, at the Grand Duke's prompting, that enabled Baden-Baden to ride the wave of fashion that was spreading across Europe at the beginning of the century. State revenues could prove a life and death matter for spas. Wiesbaden and Ems, for example, which enjoyed the sponsorship of the Duke of Nassau, grew in a fashion similar to Baden-Baden. On the other hand, spas without this support lost their viability. Such was the case with Pyrmont, located in the nearly bankrupt North-German principality of Waldeck, which, although popular in the eighteenth century, could not muster the funds necessary to remain competitive, and thus fell into a long period of gradual decline.[9]

Precisely why this state sponsorship began is difficult to ascertain, but a desire for enhanced status is a discernible feature in most cases. Each of the states in which these spas were located grew in size and standing under Napoleonic influence, their rulers rising in status. The Margrave of Baden became the Elector with the augmentation of his territory in 1805, and rose again in 1806, when he assumed the new title of the Grand Duke of Baden. Similarly, the Count of Nassau ruled over new territory and became the Duke of Nassau. Both Wiesbaden and Baden-Baden became ducal residences, in the case of Nassau, the capital, and in Baden, the summer residence near the capital of Karlsruhe. Following the pattern established in the eighteenth century, having a stylish, deluxe spa that drew prominent visitors was regarded as an item of sovereign prestige. In all likelihood, these newly elevated territorial rulers, often insecure in their recent good

[9] Although Pyrmont did not disappear, as the century proceeded, it lost its preeminent position and did not attract the kinds of numbers that were seen in Baden-Baden or Wiesbaden. For example, in 1845, Baden-Baden hosted ten times as many visitors (30,986) as Pyrmont (3,325), a number which Baden-Baden reached already in 1812; by 1865 the figures were 51,148 and 6,446 respectively. See Reinhold Kuhnert, *Urbanität auf dem Lande* (Göttingen: Vanderbroeck & Ruprecht, 1984), 57 and Heikki Lempa, "The Spa: Emotional Economy and Social Classes in Nineteenth-Century Pyrmont" *Central European History* 35, no. 1 (2002): 37-73, especially 48-51; for a complete listing of visitor statistics in the nineteenth century, see Loeser, *Geschichte der Stadt Baden*, 429. These statistics for the entire century, available intact in the archives at the end of the nineteenth century, have only survived in fragments to the beginning of the twenty-first.

fortune, found that enhancing the existing installations was a wise investment. Such places, drawing the rich and powerful, could only serve to heighten the standing of their capital cities, and by extension, the prince's own prestige.

Whatever the motivation, the Badenese government efforts to improve and promote the spa were formally institutionalized in 1805, with the establishment of the *Bäderkomission*, or Spa Commission. A department of the Ministry of the Interior, this entity was charged with the responsibility for the preservation, improvement, and promotion of the spa facilities. Part of its mission was to raise the standing of Baden-Baden vis à vis competing establishments and to ensure its financial success as an enterprise.[10] Various interests came together in this commission. Ministerial officials and members of the Badenese Senate represented the state and fiscal interest; the *Landphysicus* (a physician in a position analogous to a minister of health) and the sanitary commissioner spoke for the medical community; the well-known architect Friedrich Weinbrenner gave shape to the new improvements. Of symbolic importance, neither the mayor of the town nor any local city officials sat as members of the commission. This decision made it clear to all that the promotion and administration of the spa was a *state* interest, superseding any local considerations. For the next six decades, the administration of the spa remained separate from that of the city. The commission wielded sovereign authority on all matters of spa development, a fact of life that frequently led to friction between the state government and the local city council, which complained of having been sidelined. The priority of the government in Karlsruhe was the development of the spa, and not the wishes or well-being of the local population.[11]

---

[10] GLAKa 195/294, "Bestellung der Badekomission und deren Wirksamkeit zur Emporbringung des Bades. 1805-1808," Memorandum on the formation of the commission, August 28, 1805.

[11] GLAKa 195/294. See especially the correspondence between the City Council and the Spa Commission regarding construction projects. The local population could be resistant to improvement projects from the government from the beginning in the late eighteenth century, when innkeepers were less than enthusiastic about projects to clean the town of piles of trash and manure and (more importantly) to prescribe rates and a minimum standard that guesthouses had to offer. For factually informative if analytically thin narratives of the history of Baden-Baden, see Loeser, *Geschichte der Stadt Baden*, and Rolf Gustav Haebler, *Geschichte der Stadt und des Kurortes Baden-Baden*, 2 vols. (Baden-Baden: Verlag Dr. Willy Schmidt, 1969). The new Conversation House, discussed in greater detail below, raised greater controversy and illustrates the primacy of the state interest, i.e., the interest of the spa, in such conflicts.

The Spa Commission undertook numerous projects for the improvement and promotion of the facilities. Many of its initiatives were direct responses to the perceived needs of the visiting public, with the obvious purpose of making Baden-Baden more attractive to potential visitors, and ideally, a more profitable and successful undertaking. The Commission's decisions required the approval of the Ministry of Interior, and often involved negotiations with representatives of the medical community. The decisions were not always harmoniously or easily reached; the interests of finance, medicine, and architectural design proved difficult to reconcile on more than one occasion.[12] Nevertheless, significant improvements resulted from these arrangements.

It was in this formative period, the years between 1805 and 1830, that Baden-Baden acquired the essential infrastructure which would take it from a backwater to an elegant center for genteel society, fusing medicine and leisure. These years witnessed the improvement of the private baths in guesthouses, the establishment of new luxury hotels, and the design and construction of the central fixtures of any spa: the *Conversationshaus* (Conversation House), *Kurgarten* (garden), *Trinkhalle* (pump room), steam baths, and theater.

The *Conversationshaus*, known at first as the *Promenadenhaus*, was the first of these elements to appear on the scene. An early version, built in 1765, was a simple wooden structure consisting of a central room with two wings, designed to provide guests with a central place for social gatherings handy to the gardens or promenade on the edge of town. Despite expansion in 1802, the original *Promenadenhaus* was clearly inadequate. Guests' complaints were frequent by 1805, when the *Obervogt* of Baden (a senior administrative official) noted this dissatisfaction in a report to the Spa Commission and strongly suggested that a new one be constructed.[13] The commission responded, proposing that the former Jesuit College be converted into the new Conversation House.

This plan sparked considerable controversy. Townspeople complained about the choice of location, which entailed converting a formerly religious structure in the center of town into a place of secular, and some said decadent, amusement. What was worse, this new *Conversationshaus*

---

[12] The Court Physician Wilhelm Ludwig Kölreuter, a member of the Spa Commission, for instance, had to push for several years for the construction of a new steam-bath facility, while other 'mixed-use' or entertainment projects took precedence. It was built in 1816. See Franz Heiligenthal, *Geschichte der Stadt Baden und Ihrer Bäder* (Karlsruhe: G. Braun'sche Hofbuchdruckerei, 1879).

[13] GLAKa 195/294, "Bemerkungen des Obervogts zu Baden zu nochmehreren Emporbringung den dortigen Bäder. 1805."

would include–and this was regarded in the *Obervogt*'s report as key for meeting guests' demands–a ballroom for frequent soirées. Voices among the townsfolk raised moral objections to this proposal, perhaps a bit hypocritically, since some in the town wished to thwart the designs of outsiders in the Commission, while others had their own commercial designs on the facility.[14] The local opposition could not prevail against the state-backed Spa Commission, and the Jesuit College was converted into a new *Conversationshaus* in 1808. This temporary solution, too distant from the other key facilities, was replaced in 1822–a year of major new construction–by Weinbrenner's monumental neoclassical edifice which still stands on its carefully chosen site at the edge of the spa garden.

A central node of the spa, the Conversation House hosted a wide range of amusements: a reading salon with books, newspapers, and magazines from all over Europe, concerts, elegant formal balls, as well as perhaps the most popular amusement of all, casino gambling. The last two provoked the most vociferous opposition from the local population, who feared their corrupting effect. The Spa Commission took its revenge, declaring admission to the Conversation House and the promenade to be a "*privilegum exclusivum*" of the genteel guests, denied to the locals who were so worried about the state of their moral well-being.[15]

The spa administration had a clear interest in the casino, and in 1807, pressed the police administration for the toleration of casino gambling. The Commission made its case on the basis of anticipated revenues and in the interest of making Baden-Baden competitive with other spas that allowed gaming, one of the "usual customs of a spa visit ... and the therefore justified expectations of guests." Yet the police shared, at least in part, some of the puritanism of town residents, and therefore not only supported the *priviligum exclusivum* but also insisted on isolating the wagering from "the areas where strengthening of health, the raising of spirits and quiet" were sought–i.e., away from the curative facilities.[16]

These restrictions proved no impediment to the casino's success, however. Gambling was popular among the guests and the ban on local residents largely ineffectual.[17] Regulated after 1822 by the Ministry of the

[14] Loeser, *Geschichte der Stadt Baden*, 300.

[15] GLAKa 195/294, "Bemerkungen des Obervogts zu Baden zu nochmehreren Emporbringung den dortigen Bäder. 1805."

[16] GLAKa 195/1080, Police protocol from May 20, 1807 allowing gaming during the season.

[17] GLAKa 339/954, "Vollzug der Verordnung wegen dem Hazard Spiel, insbesondere das Verbot des Spielens hiesiger Einwohner, Handwerksburschen, Studenten und anderer Personen. 1767-1864." See for example a letter from the

Interior, gaming provided major revenues for the further development of the infrastructure and administration of the spa. In the sixteen years between 1822 and 1838, the gambling concession raised 29,000 gulden annually–a substantial sum. Casino revenues exceeded the annual expenditures of the town administration,[18] and together with the *Kurtaxe*, a fee charged to guests for admission into the finer facilities, became the fiscal lifeblood of the spa. Regardless of any moral objections, gambling, housed after 1808 exclusively in the *Conversationshaus*, was an essential source of revenue, used for the daily administration and maintenance as well as to cover improvement of the spa until the end of gaming in 1872.

The *Kurgarten* and its appurtenances were essential features of the spa. The promenade, a long walking path within the garden, allowed patrons to take their constitutionals. They were developed and expanded alongside the Conversation House. Spa physicians agreed that an important part of the therapeutic effect of a spa visit was movement in fresh air and attractive surroundings. The gardens were ideal for this purpose. They allowed genteel people to have their daily exercise in a controlled environment, protected from "raw" nature, while benefiting from the outdoors. The *Promenadeordnung*,[19] set forth all the rules for this activity, establishing standards of proper conduct and decorum and providing for their enforcement by duly appointed bailiffs. Appearance and manners were emphasized, and failure to exhibit proper attire and gentlemanly behavior were cause for ejection from the grounds. The promenade thus

---

mayor's office and the city council to the Grand Ducal Police in Baden, February 1, 1820. The spa administration constantly received complaints about "improper" elements, i.e., students, journeymen, etc., in the casino, and repeatedly attempted to address the problem, apparently without much success. One must ask, given the financial interest and consistent failure of enforcement measures, how serious these in fact were.

[18] Loeser, *Geschichte der Stadt Baden*, 296-99. These funds were kept separate from the town revenues, which, according to financial records of the city, averaged 35,000 fl. annually between 1807-09, with expenses of 26,000 fl. Thus the revenue raised for the spa by the casino concession–29,000 fl.–exceeded the annual expenditures of the town itself. How much money this represented is illustrated by the fact that the entire cost of building a new wooden theater in 1805 was 1,500 gulden (fl.).

[19] GLAKa 195/1063, "Die Bad-Polzeiordnung zu Baden, 1807." The *Promenadenordnung* was part of the overall *Bad-Polizeiordnung* (Bath Police Regulations), issued in 1807 under advisement of the *Obervogt* and the medical advisor, that regulated most areas of spa life; its 255 paragraphs saw to the minutest details.

was governed by standards of behavior and dress. One was expected to act and appear either noble or bourgeois–i.e., respectable.

Under the protective umbrella of these regulations, the respectable guest could enjoy the variety of pleasures the gardens and promenade had to offer. It was the ideal place to see and be seen, for social interaction with other guests of a similar, or even superior, social stature. It was, however, also a place where in less trafficked corners romantic interests could be pursued. Illicit pleasures were to be found there as well. Under cover of darkness, for those so disposed, the promenade became a notorious place for solicitation by prostitutes, who were officially tolerated provided they were not "too imposing or improper."[20] Here, the spa was no exception in an age when in urban environments prostitution was commonplace and conspicuous,[21] allowing males to find a more or less socially acceptable outlet for their sexual desires. Although not major population centers, the open atmosphere of spa towns offered anonymity to transient guests, and likely, prostitutes, which could only have encouraged the trade. By 1900, prostitution was regulated by the police to maintain both hygiene and discreet propriety.[22] This, too, was part of the spa experience.

Art and entertainment also belonged to the spa landscape. In addition to the concerts held in the Conversation House and the gardens, the first theater, a small wooden structure, was built in 1805. The theater, like the musical performances, offered light fare, at first performed by somewhat inferior artists. As time progressed, however, the clientele grew more demanding and the quality of the performances improved. Correspondingly, a new, more permanent and stately edifice was erected along the gardens in 1822, again designed by the prolific Friedrich Weinbrenner.

---

[20] Wolf-Heino Struck, *Wiesbaden im Biedermeyer* (Wiesbaden, 1981), 47, cited in Burkhard Fuhs, *Mondäne Orte einer vornehmen Gesellschaft* (Hildesheim: Georg Olms Verlag, 1992), 241.

[21] Richard J. Evans, "Prostitution, State and Society in Imperial Germany," *Past and Present* 70 (February, 1976): 106.

[22] GLAKa 339/1421 "Beschwerden über Dirnen," and 1422, "Überwachung der Dirnen." Complaints were usually filed by local residents, not visitors, and prostitution was evidently tolerated. The police notes to a 1907 complaint by a local resident, for example, evince a quite dismissive tone, and a letter from the City Council to the *Bezirksamt* from June 6, 1916 indicates that only when there was a severe burden, i.e., when bordellos were too overt in a neighborhood where families live, should action be taken, and they would otherwise be tolerated. A police officer noted on the back of this letter that in 1904, the city council had supported the continued toleration of this medically regulated brothel.

Alongside the amusements in the spa, the curative infrastructure occupied a place of at least equal importance. The most significant of these health facilities was the *Trinkhalle* or pump room for the morning ritual of drinking mineral water, a central steam bath facility, as well as bathing facilities in private guesthouses. These key elements were improved in order to make Baden-Baden more competitive medicinally as well as recreationally. The first *Trinkhalle* appeared in Baden-Baden in 1804. It housed one of the main sources of mineral water in the town, where guests consumed it each morning according to a well-established ritual, as was the case in spas everywhere. In Baden-Baden, it first shared a roof with the Hall of Antiquities, built to showcase the recently uncovered artifacts from the town's Roman past. Housing these two together in one impressive neoclassical edifice demonstrated the importance of water, and drinking it, as well as the imagined continuity with the Roman past. In 1822, the same year Weinbrenner's *Conversationshaus* was built, a new and expanded *Trinkhalle* was erected opposite the older structure, this time more purposefully devoted to the ritual drinking of water, with the ancient relics included almost as an afterthought.

Central steam baths also figured prominently in the modernizing spa. An old public bath, the poor bath or *Armenbad* was demolished in 1812, to be replaced in 1816 by a new facility, which in turn was expanded in 1819. After the old structure was torn down, its clientele was hustled off to a more distant location, finally in 1830 into an old medieval guesthouse. The official justification, that the *Armenbad* was decrepit and much in need of replacement, rang hollow.[23] More plausible is the explanation that the impoverished and unsightly patients of the poor bath were upsetting incongruities in the refined atmosphere of the curing district, and had to be removed in an act of gentrification.

The Spa Commission clearly put the comfort of respectable guests before the well-being of the poor. As one guidebook approvingly described it, the police endeavored to "carefully remove beggars, repulsive and disgusting objects ... for the comfort of visitors."[24] A letter of June 1810 from a local publisher to the Ministry of the Interior illustrates the general attitude toward the less affluent. A directive from the local authorities ordered that only rich and respectable visitors were to be included in the published list of guests, because no one would care about

---

[23] GLAKa 195/1032, "Die Verlegung des Armenbades und die Verbindung desselben mit dem Pfründner-Hospital (Geh.Rat) 1806-1807."

[24] G.C.W. Rullmann, *Wiesbaden und seine Heilquellen für Curgäste beschrieben* (Wiesbaden: Ludwig Schellenberg, Hofbuchhändler und Hofbuchdrucker, 1823), 46.

the others. The ministry responded, directing that all paying guests should be listed by name, but that those in the *Armenbad*–the poorest–would only be listed by number.[25] Ability to pay, then, was the entree to the official lists of respectable guests, a recognition of one's status in the world of the spa. The poorest visitors were segregated spatially and conceptually in the lists from the more wealthy and respectable–a pattern that continued in many forms throughout the nineteenth century and one that leaves no doubt about the class basis of the spa.

The new steam baths were expensive and posh, with twelve private bathing cabinets on two floors, heated rooms for rest that offered all the "necessary comforts."[26] The baths were kept clean and in order by attendants on duty year round. A guest could ask their assistance in preparing "every type of steam bath according to a physician's orders" or, if so desired, the guest could take a bath without this help.[27] Tailored to the designs of the medical members of the Spa Commission, who were instrumental in its construction, this represented a state-of-the-art facility for its day. Baden-Baden, as part of the plan to promote the spa, was to be second to none in its curative function.

Yet it was not only the public amenities which fell under the watchful eye of the spa administration. The baths in private hotels and guesthouses also came under the scrutiny of the Commission. These places were where guests spent much of their time; their improvement was given priority, and here the hand of the state was seen intervening in private interest. In the first decade of the century, Baden-Baden had a large number of guesthouses, most of which were small establishments renting out a few rooms to visitors. The Commission's attention was focused on the larger establishments that could accommodate more guests and contained bathtubs for therapeutic use. Here, the emphasis was on comfort. Several of these larger guesthouses, such as the *Salmen* (Salmon), *Sonne* (Sun) and *Baldreich* dated back at least to the seventeenth century, appearing in a 1625 description of the town's bathing establishments.[28] These were now

---

[25] GLAKa 195/1065. "Badlisten bzw. Verzeichnisse über die in Baden sich aufhaltenden Fremden (Badgäste) 1810." Letter from *Amtsmann* Schnitzler to the Ministry of the Interior, Police Department from June 28,1810; response from the Ministry, dated August 15, 1810.

[26] Wilhelm Ludwig Kölreuter, *Die Mineralquellen im Großherzogthum Baden*. (Carlsruhe und Baden: D.R. Marx'sche Buchhandlung, 1820).

[27] Kölreuter, *Die Mineralquellen im Großherzogthum Baden*, 53.

[28] Johann Mattäus, *de Thermis Marchio-Badensibus*, (Strassburg, 1618) excerpted with some linguistic modernization from a 1625 copy in Heiligenthal, *Geschichte der Stadt Baden und Ihrer Bäder*, 51-55.

deemed clearly inadequate for the new curing public, with respectable guests having to cross the street in their bathrobes to reach run-down baths.[29] Efforts were made to encourage the proprietors to upgrade their establishments, which included regular police inspections, but these apparently met with resistance. Only marginal improvements had resulted until an ordinance in 1827 dictated a unified standard for private baths and, importantly, provided innkeepers with funds for these efforts.[30]

For all the pressure put on the older guesthouses by the administration, competition from newly built hotels that better suited the expectations of a discerning public produced better results. New construction began in the first decades of the century, for example with the Hotel *Germania*, built in 1813, which became one of the most attractive guesthouses hosting prominent guests,[31] and the *Badischer Hof*, which was the most elaborate and complete spa hotel of its time in Baden-Baden. This competition grew more fierce after 1830, when new hotels proliferated along the newly built promenade.

The *Badischer Hof* was an enterprise of Johann Friedrich Cotta, Goethe's publisher and the most important German publisher of his time.[32] Cotta, together with his partner Johann Ludwig Klüber engaged the architect Weinbrenner in 1807 to convert a former Capuchin monastery into a posh hotel offering first class rooms in a variety of price ranges, private bathing facilities, a fine restaurant, ballroom, and of course, a bookstore for the reading public. The project was only partially successful: the hotel achieved the intended high standards but produced only a modest return on the investment. Its failure as a business venture lay in several factors. The structure itself, elegant and refined, was expensive to maintain, and was ahead of its time in 1808, too large for the still relatively small high-end hotel market. By 1830, when the now discouraged and personally divided investors sold the property, market demand was great enough to sustain such enterprises; the hotel became a successful enterprise,

---

[29]GLAKa 195/294, "Bemerkungen des Obervogts zu Baden zu nochmehreren? Emporbringung den dortigen Bäder. 1805."

[30] GLAKa 195/988, "Öffentliche Badeanstalten und Generalberichte über den hiesigen Kurort, Badanstalten-Comission, 1826-1847," see especially "Bericht des Geheimen Hofrats Dr. Krammer, October, 1827."

[31] Loeser, *Geschichte der Stadt Baden*, 562.

[32] Bernhard Fischer, *Der Badische Hof 1807-1830. Cottas Hotel in Baden-Baden.* Marbacher Magazin, No. 79/1997 (Marbach am Neckar: Deutsche Schillergesellschaft, 1997), 2. See also Daniel Moran, *Toward the Century of Words: Johann Cotta and the Politics of the Public Realm in Germany, 1795-1832* (Berkeley: University of California Press, 1990).

and several new ones offering a similar level of comfort and service soon appeared in Baden-Baden. In a sense, the *Badischer Hof* anticipated the needs of the curing public before these had fully developed in Baden-Baden.[33]

From the beginning of the Commission's efforts in 1805, the primary consideration was to improve conditions to meet the expectations of a sophisticated public. Concrete responses, as in the case of the Conversation House, followed complaints of shortcomings that came from guests. Not only bureaucrats, but physicians, too, were part of this formative process. They were not always successful in realizing their goals but they made their influence felt, particularly in the overtly medical parts of the spa. The modification of the curative features of the spa was their work, and not simply a response to the consumers of services. This complex interplay of interests led in the period from 1805 to 1822 to the creation of the essential elements of the spa in Baden-Baden, which helped ensure the town's success as an enterprise and earn it an international reputation.

Similar efforts were undertaken in other spas that were Baden-Baden's main rivals in the nineteenth century. Wiesbaden and Ems also improved their infrastructure with state sponsorship during the first decades of the century. Wiesbaden constructed a new Conversation House after 1807 with state funding,[34] and expanded the gardens and medical facilities. Pyrmont struggled in vain to maintain its position of prominence through a belated and apparently inadequate improvement of its infrastructure.[35] Other spas, such as the entirely new, privately-developed seaside resort of Zoppot near Danzig, established in a Kashubian fishing village in 1823 by a private entrepreneur and physician, followed this pattern in its development. A different sort of spa, using heated sea water from the Baltic rather than thermal mineral water, Zoppot showed the common elements of a Conversation House, a garden with a promenade, as well as then state-of-the-art bathing facilities. These were key features of any spa wishing to compete for cultivated travelers seeking a cure.

Infrastructure development, while not identical, took on a similar form in various spas. The case study of Baden-Baden is emblematic of a larger pattern. Generally, spas that were successful enjoyed substantial state support, particularly in building the facilities that were key for meeting visitors expectations, offering a range of first-class accommodations, and

---

[33] Fischer, *Der Badische Hof*, 85-90.
[34] Fuhs, *Mondäne Orte*, 154.
[35] Lempa, "The Spa: Emotional Economy and Social Classes," 48.

medical and leisure facilities. Towns which could not muster such resources, such as Pyrmont, generally went into decline.

The infrastructure constructed in Baden-Baden, as well as in spas all over the German lands in the first decades of the nineteenth century, illustrates the priorities of the spa administration and the curing public. The importance attached to the Conversation House and the improvement of the level of comfort in private and public spaces alike makes clear that amusement, sociability, and luxury were indispensable elements of the curing experience. Visitors, it seems, expected a high standard, and administrators endeavored to accommodate them. Curing itself, however, was equally indispensable, as evidenced by the steam baths and *Trinkhalle*.

Modern observers might be inclined to dismiss this dimension of the spa, seeing the curative aspects as part of the entertainment, medical treatment of the imaginary illnesses of the rich. Yet this would be a serious misreading of the culture of the spa. Whether there were real health benefits for the consumer is not the issue. There is considerable evidence to suggest that patrons were earnest about the cure. Visitors in fact used the medical facilities in a disciplined way. Regrettably, statistics for the number of baths given in the first decades of the nineteenth either do not exist or have not survived into the twenty-first, but some indications can be found in the literature of the time. G. C. W. Rullmann, a doctor practicing in Wiesbaden, felt in 1823 that the bathing facilities were insufficient to accommodate the large number of guests, estimating that at least 60% of all who traveled to the town, including transient guests, took the waters. The concern evidenced by Baden-Baden's Spa Commission for both the private facilities and the public infrastructure–building and then rebuilding both a *Trinkhalle* and steam bath facility in the course of twenty years–illustrates their importance. If these had not been deemed essential to the spa, it is hard to imagine that the Grand Ducal government, which controlled the purse strings, would have invested so much treasure.

At first, the coexistence of curing and entertainment may appear to be in conflict. When the entertainment was gambling, this was especially the case, as the police deliberations surrounding the casino demonstrate. Games of chance, however, were viewed as a vice to be tolerated; leisurely strolls and pleasant social interaction, on the other hand, were looked upon as virtuous, healthful activities. Curing and leisure were understood as an integrated whole, with leisure activities "used in moderation represent[ing] in fact a powerful … means for healing of the sick."[36] This view,

[36] Rullmann, *Wiesbaden und seine Heilquellen*, 51.

reminiscent of Heinrich Bebel's sixteenth-century notion of the harmony of amusement and curing, was congruent with the concept of a holistic dietetics, which entailed the regulation of bodily intakes of all kinds. It was further bolstered by concepts in German Romantic medicine, as will be discussed in greater detail below.[37] In the spa, leisure and curing belonged together as part of the whole curative experience. For contemporaries, at least, they implied no contradiction.

Exclusivity was also important in the curing experience. The rules of decorum established the finer areas of the spa as an exclusive space, with clear admission criteria. The ability to pay gave access to the wealthy while simultaneously segregating the poor outside the main district. Yet it was not only a matter of money. The *Promenadenordnung* and prohibition of persons of lower standing in the casino were designed to ensure a degree of social exclusivity based not solely on wealth, but on codes of behavior, manners, and attire corresponding to those of the *Bürgertum* and its obvious role-model in all such matters, the nobility. Together with the *Kurtaxe* this helped define the spa as a space for those able to observe the social proprieties and in possession of the right degree of *Bildung*. That such an ethos could also accommodate profitability in the case of the casino and illicit pleasures in the case of a widely tolerated prostitution seems to have raised few questions from contemporaries about hypocrisy or morality.

Sparkling new buildings were, of course, important. But success required a good deal more. It may well have been "the fashion, and some would say, the proper thing to do, to travel in the summertime to spas."[38] Once there, prominent visitors, both noble and bourgeois, set the tone that others emulated. Most nineteenth-century chroniclers of spa life attributed the fashionability of a given spa in no small part to the number and station of its aristocratic visitors, who could easily be identified from the daily lists of notable guests. This was a matter of intense interest, not to the aristocrats themselves, but to the bourgeois visitors who basked in the reflected glory of their betters. So, for example, the regular visits of Grand Duke Karl and his wife, Stephanie née Beauharnais (a niece and adoptive daughter of Napoleon) beginning in 1804 or of Queen Luise of Prussia in

[37] See Lempa for a discussion of the link between "the economy of emotions" and the curative experience in "The Spa Emotional Economy and Social Classes," 43-46.
[38] GLAKa 195/1062, "Ankündigung einer neuen Wochenschrift unter dem Titel: Hygieia, oder die Nymphe von Baden." July 1807.

the same year, were emphasized as elevating the town of Baden to a resplendence and importance that few other spas enjoyed.[39]

The "quality" of these guests was visible for all to see in the *Kurliste*, or registry of more respectable guests, which were published in most spas, including Baden-Baden, beginning in the late eighteenth century. During high season (usually May through September), these lists were published more frequently, even daily; at other times of the year much less often. The lists served two purposes, as an internal memo from August 12, 1806 in the archival records for Baden-Baden indicates.[40] First, they were to facilitate guests finding each other in town, as the names were grouped by the hotel or guesthouse in which persons were staying. This would help improve the important social interaction aspect of the spa visit. Second, they broadcast the celebrity of the spa, i.e., they were a form of advertising, designed to exploit the more numerous bourgeois guests' desire to share the same space with prominent figures. Being known as a place frequented by the high and mighty was good for business, and spa administrations made much of the social standing of its patrons.

The thought of hobnobbing with nobles was one attraction at the spa, but added to the mix of luminaries were prominent literary figures as well. None other than Goethe was an avid visitor of spas throughout German lands. To this day, the lore of Baden-Baden attempts to cash in on his reputation, making much even of a visit that never actually took place (because of a broken carriage wheel en route to the resort town).[41] Other literary and artistic figures helped promote the standing of a spa by their frequent visits. Frequent guests in Baden-Baden were Ludwig Tieck, Rahel Varnhagen, Clemens Brentano, Heinrich Jung-Stilling, and Ludwig Uhland, just to name a few of the prominent Romantic literary figures who visited Baden-Baden for the season, either for leisure or as in the case of Tieck, to seek a cure for chronic gout.[42] This parade of literary figures,

---

[39] Loeser, *Geschichte der Stadt Baden*, 430. In exemplary fashion, Loeser devotes an entire section of his lengthy history to the visits of monarchs, ascribing to them a central role in the spa's prominence.

[40] GLAKa 195/1061, "Oberamtsberichte über die in Baden angekommenen und wieder abgereisten Badgäste; die Badlisten (Reg.) 1806-1808. 195, Nr. 1061," point seven of a memo dated August 12, 1806.

[41] See Haebler, *Geschichte der Stadt und des Kurortes*, 2: 64.

[42] For an extensive listing of German Romantic figures in Baden-Baden, including literary references and excerpts, see Heinrich Berl, *Baden-Baden im Zeitalter der Romantik: die literarische und musikalische Romantik des neunzehnten Jahrhunderts* (Baden-Baden: Willy Schmidt, 1981). Berl's work is sparse on analysis, but his name-dropping gives a good indication of the high regard the literary elite had for Baden-Baden in the early part of the century.

encouraged, one should note, by the publisher Cotta, contributed significantly to the reputation of the spa town as not only a stylish, but also a cultured place to be.

Public and private parties interested in the prosperity of their spa were not satisfied to rely solely on word of mouth about prominent visits to ensure success, however, and turned to promotion in a variety of publications and in the press. Travel reports from spas appeared in newspapers and periodicals, while a large number of travel guides, both medical and non-medical, advised the reading public. Nearly every spa in German lands had a guidebook published praising its particular virtues, with updated editions appearing frequently. Although they purported to provide unbiased, objective information about the ever-more popular spas, these publications were in fact advertisements produced by those with vested interests.[43]

The authors were commonly either private persons with an undisclosed commercial connection to the spa about which they were writing, or in the case of medical guidebooks, spa physicians affiliated with the administration. These parties had much to gain if their spa grew in popularity. More visitors meant more paying customers for hoteliers and physicians alike, and for those in some official capacity, it meant that they had performed their task of representing the spa's interest, and hence the state's as well.

The authors of these promotional materials painted an idealized portrait of the spa. They mentioned little of anything unpleasant unless forced to counteract negative information published elsewhere, and then they made sure to tout the fine measures that had already corrected the situation. Although transparently biased, the advertising function of these materials is useful to the historian. Telling readers what they wanted to hear, making Baden-Baden, Wiesbaden, or Ems seem to be everything a potential guest could want in a spa, may not be a precise guide to the reality of these places, but contemporary advertising reveals much about the expectations of the spa-going public. In this sense, as in the case of the construction projects undertaken, some conclusions can be drawn as to the desires of consumers, who mostly were members of the educated middle class, or *Bildungsbürgertum.*

---

[43] Examples of this kind of guidebook from this period include: Wilhelm Ludwig Kölreuter, *Die Mineralquellen in Großherzogtum Baden*, Karlsruhe and Baden, 1820; Rullmann, *Wiesbaden und seine Heilquellen*; Hartman Christian Thilenius, *Ems und seine Heilquellen für Bade- und Brunnengäste beschrieben und mit einer Anleitung zu ihren zweckmäßigen Gebrauche versehen* (Wiesbaden: Schellenberg, 1816).

The most vigorous and widely distributed promotional efforts were those produced by the private sector. Beginning in 1807, and continuing until the publication's demise in 1865, the *Morgenblatt für gebildete Stände* published so-called "correspondence reports" from Baden-Baden signed, as were most contributions, with a pseudonym.[44] It is of note that the *Morgenblatt*, a periodical which enjoyed widespread readership throughout German lands among the educated middle class, was published by none other than Cotta, co-owner of the previously mentioned *Badischer Hof*. His partner, the Heidelberg professor of law and Badenese *Staatsrat* (state counselor) Johann Ludwig Klüber, took the lead in the marketing efforts. The first of these reports, written by Klüber, appeared literally days after he and Cotta had acquired the property for the *Badischer Hof*.[45] Singing the praises of Baden-Baden, in what can be thought of as an early version of the infomercial, the author was clearly not interested in objective reporting but in drumming up business among the educated public.

The reports stressed the diverse virtues of Baden-Baden. Early on, emphasis lay on the fine new facilities for guests, highlighting those of the *Badischer Hof*, of course, in an effort to promote the image of an up-to-date spa for those with sophisticated tastes. As the reports continued to appear in the next decades, the *Morgenblatt* consistently praised what Baden-Baden had to offer. The most frequently recurring theme, related as it was to the hotel, was the comfort available to guests. Accommodations were first-class, offering private bathing rooms and individual bathtubs of polished stone for each guest in the "bath house built in the finest style."[46] The hotel, the gardens, and the Conversation House offered the highest standard available. The entertainments, excursions into the exceptionally beautiful and unspoiled nature of the Oos Valley surrounding Baden-Baden, concerts and theater performances, and elegant balls were lauded

[44] The authorship of these documents is not entirely clear. Leonard Korth, the editor of a collection of such reports from Baden-Baden from the first half of the nineteenth century, contends that they were the brainchild of Cotta himself, citing a contemporary acquaintance of the publisher. Bernhard Fischer, who studied Cotta and his hotel, the *Badische Hof*, contends that they were the creation of Cotta's partner Klüber, making clever use of Cotta's publishing resources to market Baden-Baden. In either case, these reports should be viewed critically as a form of advertisement and not as objective reports. See the introduction in Leonard Korth, ed., *Baden-Baden in der ersten Hälfte des 19. Jahrhunderts* (Baden-Baden: J. Pfeiffer, 1911) and Fischer, *Der Badische Hof*, 38.

[45] Fischer, *Der Badische Hof*, 38.

[46] *Morgenblatt for gebildete Stände* 275 (November 16, 1808), 1099 f., excerpted in Fischer, *Der Badische Hof*, 43-44.

as the finest one could find. All this combined into a grand image of luxury and refinement that attracted, so the reports averred, a large number of the best of people. The unqualified praise, the strings of superlatives, the lack of any good thing to say about the competition –all this presaged a future Advertising Age. In this, as in many other respects, the spa and its culture was cutting edge.

The *Morgenblatt* proudly reported that Baden-Baden hosted the finest of society, for this, too, was an obvious selling point for the prospective client. The paper, at times in the most egregious manner, engaged in relentless name-dropping of princely visitors. Yet it would not do to go too far in this direction. The most numerous guests would be bourgeois in origin; they might be too easily intimidated by the presence of too many illustrious noblemen. To counter this possible danger, and to entice this particular middle-class clientele, the notion of "spa freedom" or *Kurfreiheit* was adroitly brought into play. In the bracing atmosphere of the spa, all respectable people could come together, if not as equals, then certainly in a shared conviviality that placed, at least for a while, less emphasis on caste and class. As the *Morgenblatt* formula would have it, this was a veritable bourgeois paradise, where "every difference of status disappears, a true equality emerges, and yet nowhere is a sense of respect injured."[47] "Democracy" without the rancorous intrusions of the lower class, without tawdry politics of any kind, was so much tidier than the radical and revolutionary stirrings of the world outside the spa.

The medical value of Baden-Baden was also a favored subject in the *Morgenblatt*. Scientific descriptions of the waters would interest the educated general reader, and could serve to support the claims of the healthful effects of the spa. Nonetheless, a sort of damage control was necessary to counter the "baseless" claims made even by "experienced physicians" that the waters of the Taunus or Bohemian mountains (i.e., Wiesbaden and Karlsbad) were more effective than those found in Baden-Baden. As one report in 1822 argued, the "variety of natural remedies" found in the Oos Valley spa, including the waters themselves and the sophisticated manner of their use, in conjunction with the surrounding nature and pure air made Baden-Baden "the most excellent of German spas."[48] This competition between spas in claims of medical efficacy continued throughout the century.

---

[47] *Morgenblatt*, (specific date and number not given, 1816), reproduced in Korth, *Baden-Baden in der ersten Hälfte des 19. Jahrhunderts*, 8.

[48] *Morgenblatt* (1822), in Korth, *Baden-Baden in der ersten Hälfte des 19. Jahrhunderts*, 18-19.

The *Morgenblatt* covered the gamut of attractions in Baden-Baden in order to appeal to all who might "seek healing, a change of air and entertainments of various kinds."[49] Klüber's other promotional projects endeavored to give the spa a more mysterious appeal. He wrote a two-volume guide to the town published in 1807 and 1810 by Cotta. The first provided its readers with little practical information other than the "purposeful and tasteful" character of the spa's facilities.[50] Klüber focused instead on the town's past. In one section he educed its Roman roots, artifacts of which had been on display since 1804 in the newly-built museum and *Trinkhalle*. Fantasizing on the basis of a few ruins and artifacts that had been uncovered, he offered a description of the Roman Aurelia Aquensis in all its splendor, with vivid descriptions of its baths and temples. On a promontory overlooking all twelve mineral springs, the site of the current ducal castle, Klüber depicted a temple to Asclepios–presumably an *Asclepeion*. Evoking a wondrous Roman past made Baden-Baden seem a fascinating place, and highlighted the importance of the waters and healing in antiquity, and by extension, Klüber's time.

Klüber invoked the medieval past as well, presenting a titillating description of the subterranean passages found beneath the castle. He painted a portrait of a frightening yet fascinating place, in his time frequently visited by guests, that earlier generations viewed with "horror" as "scented with the banished souls of the departed and goblins, with rattling creatures."[51] In his gothic descriptions of particular places, he relished retelling the legends of their purpose, from chambers containing hidden treasure to traps (perhaps still functioning?) which cruelly disemboweled intruders; after fully exploiting the medieval horrors, he dismissed the whole story as mere speculation, of course. Klüber here played into the emotional desires of potential guests. The underground passages appealed to the Romantic era's sense of mystery and danger, of the fascination with things past and subterranean, which became an extended metaphor for the soul and sexuality.[52] The Roman ruins and

---

49 *Morgenblatt* (1816), in Korth, *Baden-Baden in der ersten Hälfte des 19. Jahrhunderts*, 7.

50 Johann Ludwig Klüber, *Baden bei Rastatt, nach den unterirdischen Gängen und Kammern des Schlosses, nach den neuesten und künftigen, und nach den ehemaligen römischen öffentlichen Gebäuden und Anlagen der Stadt.* (Tübingen: Cotta'sche Buchhandlung, 1807), 45.

51 Klüber, *Baden bei Rastatt*, 7.

52 For a thought-provoking discussion of the German Romantic fascination with mines and caves, see Theodore Ziolkowski, *German Romanticism and Its Institutions* (Princeton: Princeton University Press, 1990), Chapter Two.

fanciful tale of their meaning gave the spa a claim to continuity with a distant past, the splendid baths of Aurelia Aquensis, now revived in the contemporary spa, Baden-Baden.

Private promotional efforts appealed to potential guests on several levels, from the fine amenities present in the spa, but also to the locality's ambiance, its intangible emotional appeal. Sponsored guidebooks, the form preferred by spa administrations, while not ignoring the amenities, tended to place greater emphasis on the medical efficacy of the waters and environment. This should come as no surprise, since the authors of most of these guidebooks were spa physicians. Despite all the amusements and comfort in the spa, they insisted, curing was the prime rationale for its existence. Many visitors came not for entertainment, but for healing, often acting on a medical referral. Therefore, doctors and potential patients were an important audience for advertising that could not be neglected.

This being the case, these guides are an important source of evidence concerning the medical knowledge and theory of the period. German Romantic medicine at the beginning of the nineteenth century tended to see the patient holistically, in his or her emotional and physical entirety. These two were regarded as integral parts of a patient's totality. The natural philosophy of Friedrich Wilhelm Schelling was notably influential in German medicine of the period, especially in southern German lands.[53] A key figure in German Romantic medicine, Andreas Röschlaub, a personal friend of Schelling, proved to be a tireless promoter of an integrated theory of medicine.[54] His system took into account the whole patient, moving beyond pure empirical observation and into an ideal world which transcended what was materially observable. In this realm, theoretical speculation reached beyond the limits of experimental science and led to a more profound truth about nature, disease, and the underlying causes of suffering. In practice this meant seeking a complex understanding of all factors contributing to pathology. The goal of therapy was to counteract external pathogenic factors, creating in effect a new, healthful environment which would then guide a person back to health.[55]

The influence of this school of thought was apparent, one might even say, made to order, for spa medicine of the early to mid-nineteenth

---

[53] Wolfgang U. Eckart, *Geschichte der Medizin*. 3rd ed. (Berlin: Springer, 1998), 264.

[54] Röschlaub, an academically trained physician, championed his views in journals he published himself. See Günter B. Risse, "Philosophical' Medicine in Nineteenth-Century Germany: An Episode in the Relations between Philosophy and Medicine." *Journal of Medicine and Philosophy* 1, no. 1 (1976): 82.

[55] Risse, "Philosophical' Medicine," 81-82.

century.[56] Seen as a product of the inner life of the earth, indeed, of primordial life itself,[57] water was an important therapeutic medium in German Romantic medicine. Drawing on the concept of a unity between the natural and the spiritual, or ideal worlds, spa medicine rested to a large degree on the curative properties of the waters themselves. Each source contained a particular invisible spirit or *Brunnengeist*, which became manifest in the healing properties of the waters.[58] A patient drinking these waters would be linked mysteriously to all of nature and universal life.[59] Of course, these waters, being so potent, could not be taken frivolously, and had to be applied properly in order to ensure a successful treatment.

These guides were written by university trained physicians for an audience of other physicians, who might be considering sending a patient for a curative, and for potential spa guests themselves. A few were written by physicians for the general public. The authors were frequently spa doctors, often with an official capacity at a given spa. So, for example, the court physician (*Hofmedikus*) of Baden was the editor of an 1820 guide to the mineral waters of the Grand Duchy for physicians and patients.[60] The medical counselor (*Medizinalrat*) of Wiesbaden, a balneologist often cited in other guides, wrote a guide to Wiesbaden for spa visitors in 1823.[61]

What may appear to modern eyes as a blatant conflict of interest caused little comment at the time. The authors' perspective is clearly that of a practicing physician with a vested interest in promoting his spa. Because the doctors often were acting in an official capacity, producing works commissioned by the spa administration, this parallel interest is represented as well. How this worked can be seen in materials concerning Baden-Baden. Internal correspondence reveals that the Badenese Sanitary Commission of the Ministry of the Interior began collecting reports about the efficacy of the waters and therapies in 1817 from practicing

---

56 Annette Drees, *Die Ärzte auf dem Weg zu Prestige und Wohlstand. Sozialgeschichte der württembergischen Ärzte im 19. Jahrhundert* (Münster: Coppenrath, 1988), 278.

57 Edith Heischkel, "Das Wasser als Arznei in der romantischen Medizin." *Sudhoffs Archiv für Geschichte der Medizin und der Naturwissenschaften* 36 (1952): 130.

58 Johannes Steudel, "Geschichte der Bäder- und Klimaheilkunde" in Walther Amelung and Arrien Evers, eds. *Handbuch der Bäder- und Klimaheilkunde* (Stuttgart: Schattauer, 1962), 16.

59 Heischkel, "Das Wasser als Arznei," 130.

60 Kölreuter, *Die Mineralquellen in Großherzogtum Baden.*

61 Rullmann, *Wiesbaden und seine Heilquellen.*

physicians.[62] Reports from practitioners then appeared in Kölreuter's 1820 guide. A later study of the efficacy of the waters commissioned by the Sanitary Commission in 1823 appeared in condensed form as advertisement to counter unspecified "misconceptions" in Paris in 1824,[63] and then as a guide in 1830.[64] Given the similar government interest in promotion and development in other spas, such as Wiesbaden, and the offices and titles of most guidebook authors of the period, it is safe to conclude that Baden was not unique in commissioning this kind of publication. The resulting guidebooks and treatises were important forms of advertising and promotion in this period that achieved some of their credibility because they also claimed to be scientifically objective.

The Badenese Kölreuter was clear about his motives for assembling his guide. The first sentence states that the "purpose of this work should be first to more closely acquaint physicians and their patients in the fatherland as well as abroad with the nature, healing properties and medical facilities of our own [Badenese] waters, which at the time have not received the honor they deserve."[65] His further goal was to counter the trend in which physicians sent their patients to popular, yet distant foreign spas, attracting them rather to closer, i.e., Badenese, spas through "unbiased" information and knowledge.[66]

Kölreuter emphasized several elements to make Baden-Baden especially attractive to potential visitors and to the physicians who prescribed taking the waters to patients. The new state-of-the-art facilities and their fastidious cleanliness were in the spotlight, as well as the extraordinary efforts the administration undertook to ensure their medically correct and attentive operation. Exacting accounts of the facilities and their use, including illustrations, impressed the reader with the sophistication of Baden-Baden. The emphasis throughout was the medical effectiveness of the treatments, in terms and language directed

---

[62] GLAKa 195/979, "Berichte des Physikats über die beobachteten Wirkungen des Badwassers bei Krankheitsfällen; sowie die Veröffentlichungen in französischen Blättern über die Eigenschaften und Wirkungen der Heilquellen, 1817-1827."

[63] GLAKa 195/979, Letter and translation into French from Dr. W. Kramer to the Sanitary Commission of the Ministry of the Interior, January 23, 1824, see also a memo from January 9, 1827.

[64] [first name not given] Kramer, *Ueber die Eigenschaften, Wirkungen, und den zweckmäßigen Gebrauch der warmen Mineralquelle so wie der natürlichen Stahlbäder zu Baden in Großherzogthume* (Karlsruhe und Baden: Marx'sche Buch- und Kunsthandlung, 1830).

[65] Kölreuter, *Ueber die Eigenschaften*, p. i.

[66] Kölreuter, *Ueber die Eigenschaften*, p. iii.

toward physicians with occasional explanations directed toward the layman.

Guides written by physicians for a more general public, such as one by the Wiesbaden Medical Counselor (*Medicinalrat*) Rullmann, offered information that clearly took the audience into consideration.[67] The initial chapters of this guide gave rich descriptions of the facilities, available at any price range to accommodate any budget, from the opulent to the relatively modest. In addition, all the pleasant diversions appeared in appealing detail. One reads of the romantic walking paths surrounding the spa, of the promenade, the delightful and well-appointed coffee house in the Conversation House; all of which enticed potential visitors interested presumably in more than simply a healthful retreat. Nevertheless, this guide like all the others concurred with Rullmann that these diversions could be a good and healthful part of a curative, when taken in moderation and under the supervision of a physician.

Regardless of the intended audience, each of the physicians writing guides to the spas was clearly interested in promoting the proper and healthful use of the bathing establishments. They all agreed: "proper use" absolutely required following a physician's expert advice. Kölreuter emphasized throughout his guide that in order to ensure a felicitous outcome of any treatment of taking the waters, be it a steam, immersion, or drinking curative, a patient must scrupulously follow a physician's orders. Long segments of his work presented the case notes of several spa physicians, the same that had been requested by the Sanitary Commission, that described successful cures of a range of maladies, from gout and rheumatism, malaise and hypochondria, through several critically ill individuals saved through the proper application of the therapies in Baden. After praising these successful cures, he warned of the ill effects that could befall people carelessly disregarding their doctor's recommendations, or worse, frivolously taking the waters on their own without appropriate guidance. An otherwise healthy person could suffer adverse effects by improper use of the powerful waters, and those already ill could face greater complication of their maladies. The only sensible and safe way to take the waters, and indeed, to behave in the spa, Kölreuter contended, was by closely following the recommendations of one's doctor. This view was echoed in many guides, sometimes more intimidatingly, as when Zwierlein threatened those foolish enough to take the waters lightly, without proper cause or direction, with potentially lethal consequences.[68]

---

[67] Rullmann, *Wiesbaden und seine Heilquellen*.

[68] Zwierlein, *Ueber die neuesten Badeanstalten in Deutschland*, 79-80.

Rullmann, admonished his more general readers that the main reason why any spa visitor would not experience the healing effects of the waters was his or her own irresponsibility. While recognizing a person's own responsibility for his or her own health, the Wiesbaden Medical Counselor stressed that the visitor himself could not be trusted with too much information or autonomy. If a cure-seeking person were handed too much information, he argued, "he would only misuse it; he would, to the great endangerment of his health ... try to be his own doctor."[69] He concluded, just as Kölreuter did, that the most important rule for a person to follow before, during, and even after a spa visit, was to seek a physician's advice and to "follow it precisely."[70]

Rullmann, also like Kölreuter, did not restrict his notion of the required compliance to a physician's instructions merely to the manner in which a guest took the waters, but extended it rather to a person's entire sojourn. The ill effects of bathing or drinking mineral water in an improper fashion could be further complicated by distraction. Essential for any cure to be truly effective was a calm and peaceful environment. Above all, a cure-seeking visitor was to avoid any sort of over-stimulation, be it through excitement, agitation with the affairs of everyday life, or equally as dangerous, overindulgence in the diversions of the spa. Excesses of wine and victuals, late-night gaieties in the theater or ballroom, and worst of all casino gaming all would scuttle any curative effect the waters might have, even in a properly applied treatment regimen. If a physician's expert therapy failed, then, it was solely the patients' own fault.

Clearly, each of the physician authors felt that expert medical advice was indispensable to successful treatment at the spa. The powers of the waters were simply too great to be entrusted to the uninitiated, who could recklessly endanger themselves by not scrupulously following a physician's advice. Yet in the authors' repeated admonitions to patients not to attempt self-treatment, as well as in direct complaints that "often a large number of spa guests" take the waters without a doctor's advice,[71] it is clear that patient compliance was far from universal, or that many spa visitors did not seek medical counsel at all. Medicine played an important role in the spa, as the construction of new bathing facilities and their place in private, non-medical advertising suggests, but curing was not necessarily undertaken under the careful direction of a physician. Given the relatively limited environment and the compact availability of sources, this early episode in the struggle to establish the authority of the physician

[69] Rullmann, *Wiesbaden und seine Heilquellen*, 225.
[70] Rullmann, *Wiesbaden und seine Heilquellen*, 226.
[71] Kölreuter, *Ueber die Eigenschaften*, 95

–an important step in the professionalization of medicine –can be seen with particular clarity in the context of the spa.

Not all physicians, it must be noted, were agreed on the usefulness of the therapy offered in the chic spas. One such individual, Ludwig Julius Kaspar Mende, was alarmed by the ever-increasing number of hard working middle-class visitors to spas who in his view fell prey to the "charlatan deceptions" of spa doctors.[72] Particularly those truly ill stood to suffer the most, he argued, as they were gullible enough to trust the wild claims of wondrous cures espoused in guidebooks written by physicians. That the rich squandered their money at spas did not disturb him, but he condemned those "devilish" physicians who "enticed those, who [could] never hope for improvement of their condition, [and] deceived them with impossible hopes."[73] The truly ill, he counseled, should save their money and health and avoid the spa altogether.

The growing number of visitors and apparent use of the waters suggest that Mende's plea was in vain. Thousands flocked to the spas, where a large number took the waters. This did not mean, however, that doctors of medicine could exercise their authority uncontested. On the most basic level, they could not escape the evidence that they were often unsuccessful. Two hundred years ago, to a much greater extent than today, many patients, despite the best efforts of their doctors, could not be healed. The medical spa guidebook authors' attempt to deal with this reality reveals much about their situation. They appear supremely confident in themselves and their waters. Any therapeutic failure they generally blamed on the non-compliant patient, rather than any real limitation of their art. One suspects, however, that blaming the patient for failed therapies was a contrivance of physicians to obscure the real limitations in their abilities, escape responsibility, and bolster their own authority. In reality, however, even a university trained doctor of medicine at this early stage of scientific medical practice had little more to offer beyond comforting words; perhaps his training would yield an accurate diagnosis, but the treatments at his disposal were usually ineffective and sometimes deadly. In objective terms, he was little or no better than that of lay practitioners like midwives

[72] Ludwig Julius Kaspar Mende, "Ueber den Besuch der Bäder und den Nutzen der Mineralwasser" *Monatsschrift für Deutsche* 2 (1801): 114. Mende was clearly a university-trained physician, having published a handbook on forensic medicine 1819, and one work on Luther and celibacy in 1818, in Latin. Accessed electronically from the University of Bielefeld electronic collections on December 20, 2002 at www.ub.uni-bielefeld.de/ digibib.aufkl.html.

[73] Mende, "Ueber den Besuch der Bäder," 115.

and herbalists.[74] His claims to unquestioned authority could not have carried much weight, hence the insistent stridency of the guidebooks.

Division within the ranks, as Mende's critique of his spa colleagues reveals, was one of the obstacles to the achievement of medical authority early in the century. Competing claims, diverse training and qualifications, not to mention approaches to medicine, all hindered physicians' efforts to establish themselves as experts to be trusted in questions of health.[75] It was, however, authority based on their putative expertise that they claimed. As the keepers of the secret knowledge of science and nature, they claimed and felt that they deserved unconditional obedience and respect from educated laypersons who may have understood some things, but did not comprehend the arcane arts of healing, and were well advised not to tamper with forces beyond their ken. Physicians, on the other hand, were initiates in the arts, experts of the field, and thus authorities to be trusted and followed. In the spa, as they would have it, a doctor's word was a "decree" (*Machtspruch)* to be obeyed.[76] That these principles were so strongly and repeatedly expressed betrays a degree of insecurity. Possession of respect and authority was the wish; the reality was less perfect. This, too, is reflected in the spa literature. Doctors still depended on patients' fees and patients, unfortunately, had to be catered to. While emphasizing that the only wise use of the waters was under medical direction, the doctor-authors undercut their own authority by providing bathers with a wealth of detailed instructions for the proper and safe implementation of the cure. Complain though they might of patients flaunting their advice, still they were the ones who felt compelled to enable them to do precisely that.

As physicians would have it, they were experts to be trusted. Yet their own words reveal a conflict with their patients. An examination of the writings of patients during this period provides a necessary corrective view to the struggle taking place within the confines of the spa. Their experiences and perceptions, often diametrically opposed to that of the physician –and also often corroborating them from a slightly different angle of vision –are revealing but difficult to obtain. An ideal source

---

[74] Calixte Hudemann-Simon, *Die Eroberung der Gesundheit, 1750-1900*, trans. from French into German by Andrea van Dülmen. (Frankfurt: Fischer, 2000), 77.

[75] See Arleen Tuchman, *Science, Medicine and the State in Germany. The Case of Baden, 1815-1871* (New York, Oxford: Oxford University Press, 1993); also Hudemann-Simon, *Die Eroberung der Gesundheit*, 43 ff.

[76] Conrad Meyer-Hofmeister, Travel Account from Bad Bockelt, 1829, cited in Christoph Mörgeli, ed., *Europas Medizin im Biedermeyer* (Basel: Schwalbe, 1997), 306. Meyer-Hofmeister himself was a physician practicing in Zurich.

would be a number of private diaries, but these do not seem to exist. The next best alternative is to examine a combination of disinterested travel guides, written by people with no apparent vested interest in spa promotion, letters by spa visitors, and the literary descriptions of contemporary fiction, in which the spa figured as a regular subject. These will have to serve to bring to life the experience of spa visitors.

In the early decades of the century, daily life in the spa was, as a rule, a composite of curing and amusement, rather similar to the portrayal offered in non-medical travel guides. A typical day began between five and seven in the morning in the *Trinkhalle*, before breakfast or coffee, where the visitor would take between four and six glasses of malodorous, ill-flavored mineral water. This was followed by conversation and coffee, or for the more solitary, a quiet walk in the gardens. Later in the morning, the typical spa guest took a bath, prepared to exacting temperature specifications by a bath master, or *Bademeister*, following the orders of a spa physician for a patient's particular ailments and needs. Meals were often taken at the hotel or Conversation House. Here at the *table d'hôte* the fare was described as generously portioned and "quite favorable for gourmands."[77] The day might include an excursion out into nature, exploring the surrounding hills and forests, or perhaps even a perilous journey into the nether regions of the surrounding caves. Before the evening meal, the guest would again drink several glasses of mineral water, before considering the amusements of the evening–theatre, formal balls, or the casino.

It becomes apparent that the daily routine consisted of a combination of social interaction and ritualistic use of the spa's amenities. Taking the waters was an important element of the experience for the typical visitor. To him it was serious medicine. In an era when most medical therapy was ineffectual at best, it was something that a person could undertake actively in order to have a sense of doing at least something to promote health.[78]

Of course, the social nature of the cure cannot be dismissed as of no importance, for it was, after all, part of the cure. In addition to the waters' curative properties, the morning meeting at the *Trinkhalle* was the first opportunity of the day to meet old and make new acquaintances, to see and be seen, and simply to be present at the opening scene of the daily show. The remainder of the day followed an alternation of leisure and social interaction, supplemented by taking the waters at specified times. All this

[77] Alois Schreiber, *Le Guide du Voyage du Rhin*, L'Abbé Henry trans. Nouvelle Edition Considérablement Augmentée. (Heidelberg, 1818). [Original: *Handbuch für Reisende am Rhein*], p. 29. Schreiber's handbook appeared in at least four editions from 1805 to 1831, with translations appearing in French and English.

[78] Mörgeli, *Europas Medizin im Biedermeyer*, 166

took place in the relatively relaxed atmosphere of the spa, where a bourgeois visitor might sit at the same table with a noble, play baccarat with a baron, or encounter a princess along the promenade.

This opportunity for social interaction and amusement was an important part of a spa sojourn, one of the aspects that caused concern among the doctors because it could easily lead to excess and distraction from the serious business of curing. Evidence provided by guests occasionally reflected this tension between medicine and amusement. Daily life, as Rahel Varnhagen described it in her letters, was often a flurry of visits and social activity during the peak summer season, and rather dull in the off season, when one would be "nearly without any company."[79] She took the waters, but spending time with friends and acquaintances, at one's residence, in the Conversation House, or in the gardens are at the center of her descriptions. Curing, it seems, did not dominate her spa day.

Works of fiction make this point more strongly. A humorous work on one middle-class spa visitor's experience described in comic detail how despite his best intentions and efforts, the distractions of the spa town kept him from his original purpose–calming his nerves of hypochondria and anxiety on the recommendation of his good friend, his physician.[80] Nor was this bourgeois protagonist successful in enjoying the amusements of the spa, falling instead into a series of misadventures. He tries to experience all the spa has to offer, going to the *Trinkhalle*, indulging in a private bath, venturing to the gardens and the Conversation House, but lacking the knowledge of the intricate customs of these places and the refinement of his fellow guests, the protagonist repeatedly faces rejection, ridicule, and anxiety. He seeks escape from these pressures with an excursion into the countryside, but there too, does not fit in with the others. Finding himself alone on a trip into a cave, he is overcome by noxious gases, and wakes to delusions that he is to be eaten by cannibals. Here was a different view than that set forth in the promotional literature of the day, a nightmare visit to the spa, but in key questions it was not entirely contradictory. Aside from the obvious satiric intent, the novel

---

[79] Rahel Varnhagen, letter to Custine (No. 71) from November 1, 1818, in *Rahel Varnhagen, Briefwechsel,* Volume 4, ed. Friedhelm Kemp (Munich: Winkler Verlag, 1979), 174.

[80] Georg Christian Sponagel, *Meine viertägigen Leiden im Bade zu Pyrmont. Eine Brunnen-Lektüre.* 3rd unaltered edition (Pyrmont: Georg Uslar, 1824). The first edition of this work appeared in 1808, the second in 1814, both published by Gebrüder Hahn in Hannover.

exhibited the same tension between the "ideal" and the "real" spa to be found in the promotional literature produced by physicians.

The social world was not all that the reports of the *Morgenblatt* would lead one to believe. In contrast to the highly-touted spa freedom, his social superiors snubbed the protagonist at the *table d'hôte*, and he panicked upon seeing the bailiffs in the spa gardens, fearing that he, a simple bourgeois, did not live up to the standards of respectable dress mentioned in the posted rules. Mustering his courage, he found his way in, only to be swindled out of more of his money. His awkwardness in this refined environment even lead him into the appearance of sexual indiscretion and trouble with the police. Falling into a compromising position with a lady's maid, he found her at his mercy after she was discharged, and taking a platonic and cavalier pity on her, offered her a room at the hotel. This, too violated the rules of decorum. Responding to complaints, the police informed him that keeping a mistress was perfectly acceptable, just not at a respectable hotel, and provided him with a list of addresses where she could stay.

The moral of the story is that the entertainments of the spa were dangerous to the cure-seeking traveler, and prevented him from enjoying a successful sojourn. Only in the end, when the protagonist coincidentally met a friend who rescued him from danger, could he return to his original purpose: taking a cure according to his benevolent doctor's advice. This conclusion is strikingly similar to the warnings about the spa amusements the Wiesbaden Medical Counselor Rullmann gave his readers in 1823. Although little is known about the author, Georg Christian Sponagel, it is fair to wonder if he himself was perhaps a spa physician. Regardless of the possible didactic and hortatory motives, one sees here the key elements of the spa and their use, in essence as a spa doctor would present it. The uninformed guest may not be able to negotiate this sophisticated spa landscape, but the daily routine as appears in guidebooks is present here as well.

As discussed above, physician's guidebooks praised the healing properties of the waters, blaming any failure to cure on a person's own irresponsibility in not following medical advice. Spa visitors resisted this notion and, thereby, the authority of the physician. If spa visitors believed in the curative powers of the waters, they did not automatically subscribe to the notion that they would be rendered ineffective unless they strictly abided by the physician's regimen. A cure-seeking visitor might visit the spa for his or her health upon the recommendation of a physician at home. Perhaps a patient would follow his or her own doctor's advice, or would perhaps consult a physician at the spa for specific recommendations. No matter how much a physician might wish his advice to be followed precisely, his recommendations were just that, *recommendations*, not orders. This, too, was a source of tension between client and spa doctor.

Rahel Varnhagen reflected this tension, the product of her ability to seek several opinions instead of relying upon just one. She described an episode of gout, during which she had consulted several physicians, at spas and elsewhere, most of whom she found to be of little help. They all asked the same questions, postulated several possibilities of what could be ailing her, and seemed only to annoy her. She did apparently find one physician who could help, one who, she wrote, "clearly sees my whole nature,"[81] which suggests a practitioner working in manner inspired by Schelling's Romantic philosophy. Yet a year later she again complained that "no doctor could help [her]" who did not have a complete understanding of her body, that needed to have its balance restored.[82] The therapy which Varnhagen received from several physicians provided apparently at best palliative relief, not a cure. A person of her means and sensibilities was not likely to place absolute confidence in any doctor.

Other authors are more harshly critical of physicians, although spa physicians, presumably following the integrative natural philosophy that accorded mineral spring water an honored position, typically fared somewhat better. Jean Paul's satirical *Dr. Katzenbergers Badereise*, written in 1807 and 1808, offers a less than favorable impression of physicians.[83] The protagonist, the eponymous Dr. Katzenberger, is portrayed as a vain and combative figure, fascinated by the grotesque and the macabre. He collects and catalogues the cadavers of animals born with monstrous defects, and in an ironic play of words on his name, meaning literally, the protector of cats, dissects them alive for scientific research. He treats the poor, but this is done more to serve his own scientific curiosity about horrible diseases than out of a sense of charity or duty. He has little or no appreciation for beauty or poetry, but rather is cold, described as having a heart like an "empty intestine … [as] is always found in corpses."[84] The second physician appearing in this tale is Dr. Strykius, the spa practitioner and Katzenberger's nemesis. Strykius, in contrast, is genteel and sensitive, concerned with patients' welfare. Lest

---

[81] Rahel Varnhagen, letter to Marcus from February 20, 1814, in *Briefwechsel,* 4: 52.

[82] Rahel Varnhagen, letter to [her husband] Varnhagen from July 3, 1815, in *Briefwechsel*, 2: 310.

[83] Richter, Jean Paul Friedrich (Jean Paul), *Dr. Katzenbergers Badereise*, in *Jean Paul's sämmtliche Werke*, LI, vol. 1-3 (Berlin: Reimer, 1828).

[84] Jean Paul, *Dr. Katzenberger*, 2: 78.

the reader gain too favorable an impression, however, the two reconcile at the end, addressing each other in the familiar *du* when it turns out that Strykius, too, has his own collection of grotesqueries, featuring a mummified six-fingered hand.

Physicians' complaints that spa guests did not properly respect their authority are confirmed in Jean Paul's tale. In an episode in the *Trinkhalle*, a patient approached Strykius, saying "*Franchement, Mr. Médecin*, until now I have only forced down half of your prescribed glasses of this detestable stuff; I demand now that you prescribe only this half." The spa physician amicably agrees, much to Katzenberger's chagrin.[85] The patient was acting sensibly, as the author saw it. In almost a mirror image of Rullmann's view, Jean Paul suggested that taking a physician's advice too seriously could be dangerous. In one passage, Strykius comments to Katzenberger in jest, "*Bon!* Who gives life can also take it back, and you can commit murder, because you have healed often enough."[86] He repeated this view, again in jest, in another work, describing how a physician's job is ultimately to cure suffering by hastening death. The poor received worse care, dying sooner as they would be going to a better place, while the rich received better medical treatment since they would be going to Hell and should not be hurried.[87] Although humorous and satirically overstated, these views were hardly flattering to the medical profession or its lofty sense of self-esteem. Another collection of spa stories by Friedrich Laun portrayed their central figure as chronically ill, despite –or possibly as a consequence of –following his physician's advice scrupulously.[88]

An examination of sources that reflect the spa visitors' experience illustrate how the curing public in fact did not mindfully follow a physician's advice. A person might consult with several physicians, taking their recommendations with skepticism. This was justified, as the therapeutic regimens offered were not nearly as effective as the physicians' reports published in Kramer's guide to Baden-Baden would suggest. Treatment may have provided palliative relief, which physicians observed and described as success stories, but as Varnhagen's description of her chronic gout shows, illness returned. That physicians could only provide limited help, but nonetheless posed as experts, would explain spa-visitors' skepticism of physician's ability to heal their maladies.

---

[85] Jean Paul, *Dr. Katzenberger*, 2: 20.

[86] Jean Paul, *Dr. Katzenberger*, 3: 11.

[87] Jean Paul, *Auswahl aus des Teufels Papieren*. In *Jean Paul's sämmtliche Werke*, 1828.

[88] Friedrich Laun (pseud.) [Friedrich August Schulze], *Glitts Erzählungsabende im ** Bade* (Leipzig, 1821), vol. 1, p. 13.

The relative inefficacy of medical therapy is but part of the explanation of physicians' lack of authority in the early nineteenth century. In cities during the early decades of the nineteenth century, and perhaps more so in spa towns, doctors complained of the competition for patients, that the profession was simply overfilled. Academic medical practitioners had a small patient base, confined mostly to members of the educated middle class and the nobility, the kind who frequented spas, which resulted in a position of economic dependence. For members of the higher social orders, seeking medical advice was to an extent a given already in this period.[89] Contrary to the doctors' wishes, however, they were often treated by their socially superior patients as simply another servant.[90] In return, many–although certainly not all –physicians viewed their patients with contempt, expressing perhaps their resentment over their relatively weak position with complaints of ignorance and stupid comments.[91]

It seems clear that doctors of medicine did not receive the respect they felt was their due. At the same time, spa doctors, at least, attempted to assert their authority and status. This reveals more than simply economic dependence, but rather also a sense of status anxiety that was a consequence of the deterioration of the *ständisch* (caste-related) order. Into the eighteenth century, doctors of medicine enjoyed a high position in this social system, near the top of the educated caste or "*gelehrter Stand.*" In increasing measure over the course of the eighteenth and into the early nineteenth century, status based on the traditional university model gave way to the new middle-class or bourgeois conception of an educated person as not simply trained (*gelehrt*) but cultured (*gebildet*).[92] Physicians, rather than trying to create a new elite, as much of the discussion of

---

[89] Jens Lachmund and Gunnar Stolberg, *Patientenwelten. Krankheit und Medizin vom späten 18. bis zum frühen 20. Jahrhundert im Spiegel von Autobiographien.* (Opladen: Leske & Budrich, 1995), 222.

[90] This description can be found in several sources discussing the status of German doctors and the relationship with patients, see for example Claudia Huerkamp, "Ärzte und Patienten" in Alfons Labisch and Reinhard Spree, eds., *Medizinische Deutungsmacht im sozialen Wandel des 19. und 20. Jahrhunderts* (Bonn: Psychiatrie Verlag, 1989), 57-74, Lachmund and Stolberg, *Patientenwelten*, or Hudemann-Simon, *Die Eroberung der Gesundheit,* 74-105.

[91] Loetz, Francisca, *Vom Kraken zum Patienten: "Medikalisierung" und medizinische Vergesellschaftlichung am Beispiel Badens, 1750-1850* (Stuttgart: Steiner, 1993), 100.

[92] See Claudia Huerkamp, "Die preußisch-deutsche Ärzteschaft als Teil des Bildungsbürgertums" in Werner Conze and Jürgen Kocka, eds., *Bildungsbürgertum im 19. Jahrhundert, Teil 1, Bildungssystem und Professionalisierung im internationalen Vergleichen* (Stuttgart: Klett-Cotta, 1985), 358-387.

professionalization suggests, attempted to defend their position by changing with the times.[93]

Academically trained physicians occupied a tenuous position on the edge of this new educated middle class, or *Bildungsbürgertum*. A university degree in medicine did not automatically confer the status it once had in the old *ständisch* order. The new qualification of *Bildung* differentiated between the truly educated, and the "*Fachgelehrten*" (or in the pejorative, "*Brotgelehrten*" –persons trained solely to make a living).[94] *Bildung* meant more than simply education, but constituted a style of life that embraced tastes, manners, and attitudes. *Bildung* was now the ticket of entry into "good" bourgeois circles, and it was the rare doctor who held that ticket.[95] Significant gradations of status existed within the "medical brotherhood." Although some physicians did indeed enjoy a higher social standing, this was not "thanks to their medical expertise, but much more their social origin, their connections, and their general knowledge (*Allgemeinbildung*), which raised them into the ranks of the cultured (*gebildete Stände*).[96]

When portrayed in a positive light, as in Sponagel's tale, physicians were cultured gentlemen, friends, and equals. This was far from always being the case, however, as Jean Paul's image of uncouth ghoulish collectors of macabre artifacts suggests. Behind the veil of *Bildung* that some physicians might exhibit, like the spa physician Strykius, they were at heart, the Romantic author indicates, heartless and coarse, more, in fact, like Dr. Katzenberger. Jean Paul, it seems, was attempting to debunk a myth that spa physicians were somehow superior to "ordinary" uncultured physicians found elsewhere.

The manifest influence of Schelling's natural philosophy on spa medicine in this period may have contributed to a view of the spa doctor as somehow superior in that he pursued healing not as an isolated science,

---

[93] Thomas Broman, "Rethinking Professionalization: Theory, Practice and Professional Ideology in Eighteenth Century German Medicine" *Journal of Modern History* 67, no. 4 (Dec. 1995): 840.

[94] Thorsten Maentel, "Zwischen weltbürgerlicher Aufklärung und stadtbürgerlicher Emanzipation." in Dieter Hein and Andreas Schultz, eds., *Bürgerkultur im 19. Jahrhundert*. (Munich: C.H. Beck, 1996), 141.

[95] Wolfgang Kaschuba, "Deutsche Bürgerlichkeit nach 1800. Kultur als symbolische Praxis." in Jürgen Kocka, ed., *Bürgertum im 19. Jahrhundert. Band II: Wirtschaftsbürger und Bildungsbürger* (Göttingen: Vandenhock & Ruprecht, 1995), 106.

[96] Huerkamp, "Ärzte und Professionalisierung in Deutschland." *Geschichte und Gesellschaft* 6, no. 1 (1980): 351.

but rather as part of an integrated philosophy that combined nature and spirit, in harmony with the times. Advocates of natural philosophy in medicine emphasized theory and understanding in place of practical goals, more in the spirit of Romantic *Bildung* than Enlightenment utilitarianism.[97] This may have contributed to a view of spa physicians as somehow more *gebildet* and therefore more socially acceptable. At the same time, however, this natural philosophy itself served to undermine a doctor's claim to authority. If the power of healing resided in the interplay of a patient's spirit with a universal life force found in mineral waters, what essential role in this process could a physician play? Consequently, a person might seek a physician's counsel, but ultimately any cure was out of his hands. Under the best conditions, a doctor might have been regarded as a gentleman and a friend, but his authority was as of yet dubious.

Spa doctors, then, were struggling in two ways for status. On the one hand, they shared in the fight of the emerging middle class for status against the nobility. Birth and wealth should no longer be the main indicators of status, but yield to talent, knowledge, and the merit that these conferred.[98] Yet they faced the scorn of an educated middle-class society to which they only partially belonged. They vociferously, if perhaps ineffectively, asserted their authority and demanded respect as at least equals, based in contrast to the old *ständisch* order, not based on their academic title, but rather because of the knowledge, expertise, and skill they possessed. Unsuccessful at the time, this aspiration to prestige based on specialized scientific knowledge anticipates developments later in the century, when physicians would wrest from the general public the status they coveted. Although in this early period of the romantic spa one can only speak of a profession in a guarded sense, spa physicians' quest for authority with their patients illustrates an early stage in the tension between professionalization and the educated middle class.[99]

---

[97] Tuchman, *Science, Medicine and the State in Germany*, 17.

[98] For example, Christoph Wilhelm Hufeland, Goethe's physician and an influential advocate for the medicinal use of waters, was also an opponent of hereditary nobility, as illustrated by his work, *Das Adelthum im Lichte des Christenthums*. See Alfons Labisch, "Gesundheitskonzepte und Medizin im Prozeß der Zivilisation." in Labisch and Spree, *Medizinische Deutungsmacht*, 19.

[99] Werner Conze and Jürgen Kocka, "Einleitung" in Conze/Kocka, *Bildungsbürgertum im 19. Jahrhundert*, 1:25. See also the discussion of professionalization in Chapter 1.

CHAPTER FOUR

THE PRICE OF SUCCESS 1830-1870

By the early years of the 1830s, the Spa Commission of Baden-Baden could look back with considerable satisfaction at its accomplishments. In a relatively short span of time, it had succeeded in transforming the resort from a decrepit relic into a much-visited and prestigious station on the European spa circuit, frequented in ever-growing numbers by German and international society. Measured by numbers of visitors, the mid-nineteenth century, generally from 1830-1870, was a golden age for nearly all the larger spas. Baden-Baden saw the number of guests grow more than five-fold–from 8,364 guests in 1826,[1] to 33,623 in 1850, and 46,842 in 1860.[2]. By 1868, Baden-Baden reigned as the queen of German spas, hosting 56,013 visitors, nearly twice as many as the Austrian spas Karlsbad, Teplitz, and Gastein combined, and roughly double the figure for either Wiesbaden or Vichy.[3]

After 1830, a large number of visitors to the grand spas came from abroad, lending a cosmoplitan air to Ems and Wiesbaden; in Baden-Baden these years were known as the "Time of the French."[4] Baden-Baden was favored by the French and Russians, whereas Wiesbaden and Ems attracted English patrons in particular. The *lingua franca* in these cosmopolitan resorts, was of course, French, and knowledge of French was

---

[1] GLAKa 195/988, "Generalbericht über den hiesigen Kurort" for the season 1826.

[2] GLAKa 195/1232, "Herausgabe ehiner offiziellen Fremdenliste in der Stadt. Enthält: Zusammenstellungen der Fremden nach Nationalitäten geordnet. (BAKom) 1850-1866." Detailed statistics regarding visitors are compiled in annual reports in this file.

[3] Karl Frech, *Der Kurort Baden-Baden. Ein Beitrag zur Geschichte und Statistik des heutigen Badewesens* (Karlsruhe: Chr.Fr. Müller'sche Hofbuchhandlung, 1870), 35.

[4] Albert Fromherz, *Baden-Baden zur Franzosenzeit. Skizzen aus dem Badeleben vor fünfzig Jahren.* Edited and with an introduction by Karl Hauck (Baden-Baden: Peter Weber, 1905).

considered a qualification for employment in the baths. At midcentury, Baden-Baden hosted as many visitors from France as from Germany, in some years, more.[5] Middle-class Germans, however, as visitor statistics kept by spa administrations show, continued to constitute about half of the curing public. The upper-echelons of the *Bürgertum*, lawyers, higher-civil servants, and businessmen were drawn to these elite watering places by the thousands annually, often traveling considerable distances by steamship along the Rhine or by the new railroads to reach their destinations. More modest bourgeois visitors gravitated toward smaller, more affordable spas such as Schlangenbad and Wildbad in the Black Forest, and farmers and laborers, except for servants accompanying their employers, nearly disappeared from the spas.[6]

More visitors meant more business, but booming visitor statistics only tell part of the story. Although for many guests, taking the waters was eclipsed by a more important elaborate social experience, a large number continued to seek healing, or at least relief from chronic maladies. The waters themselves retained their salutary reputation with the public; in fact, faith in their ability to heal grew in the mid-nineteenth century. The same could not be said for the powers of physicians, however. By 1850, spa physicians found themselves on the defensive, striving to counter the effects of their own exaggerated claims, the rise of lay-practitioners utilizing water cures, and changes in the scientific environment, if not the curing public, that threatened to undermine faith in the waters. The mystical proclivities of Romantic natural philosophy were giving way to a more hard-headed empiricism. The spa doctors responded in various ways to this difficult situation, scrambling to maintain credibility with the middle-class public and win respect in the greater medical community. Led by a young generation, spa physicians embarked on a course which by the final decades of the century established the field of spa medicine, after the 1850s called balneology, as one with a place in academic medicine. Yet their efforts, which included professional organization and a commitment to research using modern methods, came somewhat later than

---

[5] Frech, *Der Kurort Baden-Baden*, 37.

[6] See Matthias Bitz, *Badewesen in Südwestdeutschland 1550 bis 1840. Zum Wandel von Gesellschaft und Architektur.* (Idstein: Schultz-Kirchner Verlag, 1989). Bitz' study presents analysis of the guest registries at several spas, providing valuable information, if limited critical analysis, of the social composition of the curing public. For detailed analysis of the Nassau spa town Bad Ems, see also Hermann Sommer, *Zur Kur Nach Ems. Ein Beitrag zur Geschichte der Baderise von 1830 bis 1914.* Geschichtliche Landeskunde, Bd. 48, (Franz Steiner Verlag, Stuttgart, 1999).

in other branches of medicine, and the process of gaining recognition was by no means smooth or assured. At midcentury, the authority of its practitioners was hardly unquestioned and the prospects for the specialty were not particularly auspicious. Tracing this struggle to define the essential nature of the spa and the role of its doctors through a period of critical challenges is the subject of this chapter.

The grand spas' popularity proved a mixed blessing. Many visitors came by the new railroads, which compressed time and space to make practicable a short excursion to a desirable spa, once only a dream. After 1837, the Rhine-Valley railroad conveyed visitors from distant locales to the idyllic Oos Valley in the Black Forest, where Baden-Baden was situated. Some complained that the railroads were in fact detrimental to the business climate of the town, as more mobile visitors stayed for shorter periods of time, spending less money in the end, and hurting small businesses that catered to long-term guests. Tailors, washer-women, and owners of spacious rental apartments all complained of the effects the coming of the railroad had on their revenues.[7]

The surge in the number of visitors, however, testified to how the greater elegance of these elite resorts elevated their prestige as a desirable place to be and be seen. Success raised once again the debate about the essential character of the institution. Was the spa about entertainment or was it about healing? For many, popularity tarnished the spa's reputation as havens for serious curing insofar as they appeared more as playgrounds for the idle rich than healthful resorts. Independent observers of life in Baden-Baden, Wiesbaden, and other modish resorts ranged from cautiously amused at their opulence to scathing about their decadence. For some, the self-indulgence on display rendered farcical the designation *Kurort*, place of curing.[8]

Wilhelm von Chèzy, a literary figure of modest fame and often a visitor in Baden-Baden, set down his impressions in his 1835 pocket

---

[7] "Badener Zustände" *Morgenblatt für gebildete Leser* 155, July 1, 1847, 619-620.

[8] See the various articles on spa life, such as reports from Karlsbad, Marienbad, Wiesbaden, and Baden-Baden in the *Morgenblatt*, such as "Eine Saison in Baden," *Morgenblatt für gebildete Leser* 207 (August 29, 1846): 826, 208 (August 31, 1846): 830-31; 209 (September 1, 1846): 834-35, or "Aus den Badeerinnerungen eines Hundes," *Morgenblatt für gebildete Leser* 243 (October 10, 1845): 969-70, 244 (October 11, 1845): 974-975, 245 (October 13, 1845): 978-979, 246 (October 14, 1845): 982-983, 247 (October 15, 1845): 985-986.

guidebook written for "guests seeking a curative and travelers."[9] Chèzy, without the sponsorship of the spa administration, offered a wealth of useful tips for the potential visitor. The town, he wrote, "rightly occupies one of the first places among all the most famous baths and mineral springs of Germany, owing to the recognized salubrious properties of its springs, the amenities and comforts that the guest will find there, as well as the superb beauty of the locality."[10] This brief passage encapsulated the main attractions of a spa visit: the promise of healing in a pampering and beautiful environment.

Chèzy offered the reader precise details of the waters in Baden-Baden, including the most recent chemical analyses of each spring and suggestions for further reading for those "who wish to inform themselves fully regarding the healing powers of the mineral waters in internal and external application."[11] The bulk of Chèzy's guide, however, was devoted to amusement, especially the Conversation House and the Promenade, supplemented by handy schedule and fare charts for the Rhine steamship lines and private coaches, as well as an entertaining historical sketch of the town. Chèzy's purpose, it seems, was to provide general information to a wide spectrum of visitors, no doubt because he wanted to sell as many copies as possible. Nevertheless, the guide is useful in ascertaining the popular perception of the spa near midcentury.

According to Chèzy, many came to Baden-Baden for "gaming alone."[12] This was certainly one of the prime attractions, and Chèzy, catering to his audience, devoted several pages to an explanation of the intricacies of roulette. Other authors substantiated this observation, most notably Fyodor Dostoevsky in his works *The Player* and *The Idiot*. The Russian novelist, who probably was a compulsive gambler himself, stayed in Baden-Baden and Wiesbaden several times in the 1860s, and drew on his experiences for his work. In "Roulettenburg," a thinly transparent pseudonym for Baden-Baden and Wiesbaden in *The Player*, the spa was a place of intrigue and romantic liaisons, all tainted by the lust for gold. The

[9] Wilhelm von Chèzy, *Rundgemälde von Baden-Baden, seinen Nähern und fernern Umgebungen. Ein Taschenbuch für Kurgäste und Reisende* (Karlsruhe and Baden, Marx'sche Buch- und Kunsthandlung, 1835).
[10] Chèzy, *Rundgemälde von Baden-Baden,* iii.
[11] Chèzy, *Rundgemälde von Baden-Baden,* 20. The title recommended is a medical guide written by the physician and Court Councillor Pitschaft, *Das Klima und die Heilquellen von Baden*, as well as Kramer, *Die warme Minerallquelle etc.*, 1830. These guides are of the type offering more specialized information for physicians and interested laypersons.
[12] Chèzy, *Rundgemälde von Baden-Baden,* 51.

promise of gulden, Friedrich d'or, and gold francs springing forth from the roulette wheel far outweighed the thought of mineral waters. Even visitors intending to take a curative found themselves seduced by the lure of easy riches. At first, of course, they would win. More often than not, they then squandered their new treasure greedily hazarding for more. Finally, seized by desperation, they played on into bankruptcy in a hopeless effort to recover what had been lost.[13]

German observers of the spa world also noted the malady that Dostoevsky so clearly diagnosed. Emma von Suckow, a Biedermeier author and publicist who wrote under the *nom de plume* Emma Niendorf,[14] also published her views on the Baden-Baden casino in the *Morgenblatt für Gebildete Leser* (the name updated to make it more contemporary than the earlier title, *Morgenblatt für Gebildete Stände,* in 1837). In an 1845 piece, she offered heart-rending images of women with "one common interest impressed upon their faces: disfiguring greed … as if in desperation." A "vampire for gold," a mother ignored her forlorn child, and provided only one of "all the thousand little dramas" of desperation played out daily in the Conversation House, in a "world of phantasmagoria … a universe of ephemera."[15] Illusion of riches, illusions of status all were there. It was, as noted elsewhere in the *Morgenblatt*, a place where in order to make for better appearances, "Herr Leduc from Epernay becomes *Monsieur le duc d'Epernay*, the wood dealer [*Holzhändler*] Graf became *comte* Holzhändler."[16]

The publicist and playwright August Lewald committed his opinions to paper in several 1847 numbers of the *Morgenblatt*. Lewald attempted to strike a balance between gentle disdain for the vice of gambling and its ill effects and to counter the apparently widespread perception of Baden-

---

[13] See Fyodor Dostoevsky, *The Player*, here referenced from *Gesammelte Werke in Zwanzig Bänden*. Gerhard Dudek and Michael Wegner, eds. *Der Spieler. Späte Prosa.* Trans. from Russian into German by Werner Creutziger, ed. Gerhard Dudek (Berlin and Weimar: Aufbau-Verlag, 1990), 348-530. Dostoyevski first conceived of the project in September, 1863, and completed it in 1866. See the notes to the above volume, 744-45.

[14] see Karin de la Roi-Frey, Frauenleben *im Biedermeier. Berühmte Besucherinnen bei Justinus Kerner in Weinsberg* (Leinfelden-Echterdingen: DRW-Verlag, 1998).

[15] Emma Niendorf [Emma von Suckow], "Villeggiatur in Baden," *Morgenblatt für gebildete Leser,* April 28 1845, 402-403.

[16] "Badener Zustände," *Morgenblatt für gebildete Leser,* June 29 1847, 613. These later unsigned reports could not have been the work of Johann Friedrich Cotta, as was noted in the previous chapter, given that the editor and publisher died in 1832.

Baden as a "gaming hell" (*Spielhölle*), which he clearly did not share.[17] For him, roulette was no more risky, and no more decadent, than speculation on the stock market, -which he saw equally a game of chance promising big money.[18] Others shared his view that "whist, l'Hombre, faro are child's-play. Modern gambling is the market, one can win and lose millions there. The modern gambler is the banker."[19] Those most prone to succumb to the excesses of the green table were those, Lewald stressed, already at risk, individuals already burnt out and half-dead. The shadowy characters who preyed on the unfortunate victims of the casino, frauds, swindlers, *seducteurs*, and cocottes, albeit the stuff of good tales, were in fact but small in number. Most people at the spa, the publicist asserted, were respectable "men of state, men of letters, artists, world-historical individuals, refined women, fathers and mothers with their daughters and sons."[20] Guides that emphasized the spectacular rendered a distorted picture of the truth, which he set about to correct by emphasizing the other attractions the spa had to offer. Healing waters, dramatic natural landscapes, and refined pleasures all figured prominently in these images from Baden-Baden. This, Lewald argued, was behind the scenes, so to speak, the "real" Baden-Baden. That he had to assert this point suggests that the view of the spa as a "gaming hell" was indeed prevalent, and perhaps one gaining ground with respectable middle-class people, such as composed the readership of the *Morgenblatt*.

The spa administration in Baden-Baden also recognized a problem with the casino, in much the same terms as Lewald, namely that the "wrong elements" of society were giving the spa a bad name. But it put its own class outlook to work in identifying those of presumably weaker moral fiber; the trouble-makers were journeymen, servants and students. In 1843 and 1844, the University of Heidelberg formally requested that their students not be allowed access to the casino. Between 1830 and 1850, bans were repeatedly issued on artisans, students, and all sorts of improper persons (including all without proper attire), together with reminders to the staff of the casino that these individuals were not permitted in the casino. Fines were to be levied. The repetition of these prohibitions, and the notices given to the staff, make clear that these were at best ineffectual

---

[17] August Lewald, "Bilder aus Baden-Baden" *Morgenblatt für gebildete Leser*, October 12, 1847, 975.

[18] Lewald, "Bilder aus Baden-Baden" *Morgenblatt für gebildete Leser*, October 13, 1847, 977.

[19] Heinrich Laube, "Baden," in *Heinrich Laube, Reise durch das Biedermeier*. Franz Heinrich Körber, ed. (Hamburg: Hoffmann und Campe, 1965), 280.

[20] Lewald, "Bilder aus Baden-Baden," 970.

measures, and possibly ignored outright. In 1854 the administration spelled out their position more emphatically, and evidently finally, invoking police authority to "determine which classes of persons may not be admitted to gaming."[21] In the administrators' view, something had to be done both to protect people presumably more susceptible to the seductions of gaming, and to preserve a genteel atmosphere for guests of a "better" caliber by maintaining a modicum of respectability.

Games of chance were hardly the only vice to figure prominently in the spa, however. Heinrich Laube, a newspaper editor and author counted as part of the literary movement of "Young Germany," traveled throughout German lands in 1833-37, recording his observations in a series of subsequently published travel journals.[22] His itinerary included several elegant spas, where the first sight that met him as he approached town was the throng of *filles de joie* (*Freudenmädchen*) calling to him from every window. Nor was this an isolated incident, for elsewhere young women with "eyes that had seen much," posing as musicians or servants were eager to "meet every desire."[23] Prostitution aside, the pursuit of illicit romance, the equivalent of a "shipboard romance" and renowned even today as a "cure shadow" (*Kurschatten*), dominated Laube's portrayal of spa life. Such, it seems, was also part of the much-touted "spa freedom."

The association between bathing and moral license, particularly prostitution, characterized the earlier history of the spa, as discussed in Chapter Two. Although it was not new in this period, it was apparently more widespread and difficult to control. Municipal baths had virtually disappeared from European cities by the late 1600s, in large part owing to their reputation for carousing, prurience and the resulting spread of venereal diseases, especially syphilis. In the nineteenth century, despite the complete absence of public nudity, the strict separation of the sexes, and private bathing cabinets, the association between baths and licentiousness

---

[21] GLAKa 339/954, Vollzug der Verordnung wegen dem Hazard Spiel, insbesondere das Verbot des Spielens hiesiger Einwohner, Handwerksburschen, Studenten und anderer Personen. 1767-1864, and 195/1218, "Spielordnung (-Reglement) für die Bank (BAKom), 1822-1854." Item number two of the 1854 *Spielordnung* [Gaming Regulations] specifically gave the police the authority to screen gamers by social class and appearance.

[22] Some views expressed in Laube's travel accounts were viewed as insulting to the Prussian monarchy, and resulted in the author's imprisonment. Franz Heinrich Körber, "Nachwort," in Franz Heinrich Körber, ed., *Heinrich Laube, Reise durch das Biedermeier* (Hamburg: Hoffmann und Campe, 1965), 427-434.

[23] Heinrich Laube, "Karlsbad" in *Heinrich Laube, Reise durch das Biedermeier*, 110.

remained.[24] Some critics saw little other than vice, but drew a clear link, not to the baths, but between the casino and all kinds of degeneracy. Johann Evagelist Wetzler, who published numerous popular works on medicine, wrote of the glamorous spas:

> Facilities for entertainment and amusement belong in a spa, as they can be of assistance to the spring cures. But casinos and dance balls ... are precisely the opposite. A spa is in a strict sense a place of healing. Public gaming, faro, the embodiment of everything pernicious ... truly! A public casino fits in a spa like a bordello does in a hospital![25]

In these depictions the spa appears as a place of frivolous amusement and of decadent perils for the unwary. Where, in this place ostensibly devoted to the pursuit of health, one wonders, were the sick? In the grand spas, treatment of the truly ill was eclipsed by the grand soirées, life on the promenade, and the casino. Chèzy's guide was "meant for th[e] more mobile guest, who is no stranger to the morning dew and fresh breeze."[26] The "more delicate ... the old .. the handicapped" the author suggested were not out of place but would find "comfortable and nearby cool shade, refreshing green and cheerful views"–essentially out of the way of the bustle of the more fun-loving clientele.[27] The Badenese Grand Ducal Balneologist Franz Heiligenthal conceded in his 1879 history of Baden-Baden that the sick, while present in large numbers, "moved entirely into the background" in the midcentury spa, overshadowed by those seeking amusement.[28]

---

[24] For more detailed discussion of this phenomenon, see Ernst Gerhard Eder, *Bade- und Schwimmkultur in Wien. Sozialhistorische und kulturanthropologische Untersuchungen.* Kulturstudien Bibliothek der Kulturgeschichte vol. 25, Hubert Christian Ehalt and Helmut Konrad eds. (Vienna: Böhlau Verlag, 1995), esp. 205-248.

[25] Johann Evangelist Wetzler, *Über Gesundbrunnen und Heilbäder* (Mainz, 1825), 64, 148 f., cited in Bitz, *Badewesen in Südwestdeutschland*, 324-25. Other works by the Bavarian Wetzler include *Meine wunderbare Heilung von beispielloser Hautschwäche und Geneigtheit zu Erkältungen durch eine Somnambule, mittelst Waschungen mit einer Campherseife.* 3rd expanded edition (Augsburg: Kollmann, 1844), and *Beobachtung über den Nutzen und Gebrauch des Keil'schen Magnet-electrischen rotation-Apparates in Krankenheiten* (Leipzig : K.F. Köhler, 1842).

[26] Chèzy, *Rundgemälde von Baden-Baden*, vii.

[27] Chèzy, *Rundgemälde von Baden-Baden*, viii.

[28] Franz Heiligenthal, *Geschichte der Stadt Baden und Ihrer Bäder, und Ihrer Bäder* (Karlsruhe: Braun'sche Hofbuchdruckerei, 1879), 73-74.

Obscured by frivolity, no doubt, yet still sought by large numbers of visitors, curing disappeared neither from spas generally nor from Baden-Baden, the most glittering German example. Not everyone saw the situation as grimly as the observers mentioned thus far. Eugen Guinot, in his 1858 guide for the general public, sought to correct the irresponsible view that dismissed the medicinal importance of a spa visit:

> The natural wonders of the area and the wonderful parties in Baden should not lead one to the mistaken impression that here is only a place of enjoyment and distraction; that one visits here only to find entertainment, amusement, balls and wintertime parties on beautiful summer evenings; that the mineral springs are only an excuse and no one asks for their healing powers. This is not so, and only those who know Baden by hearsay are caught in this error.[29]

Although there is no archival evidence that this particular guide, *Sommer in Baden-Baden*, was published in collaboration with the spa administration, the author so flattered the resort town that some form of sponsorship might be presumed. Regardless of any promotional motive, however, the claim that the springs were sought out for curing was in fact a valid one.

This can be seen in general travel guidebooks with no apparent vested interest, suggesting substantial interest in the waters among the traveling public. One example, the *Handbuch für Eisenbahn-Reisende durch das Grossherzogthum Baden,* published in 1842, offered general tips not only for spas, but other locations now accessible by the new and exciting railroads.[30] The reader was presented with detailed descriptions of the points of interest along the way, major cities, landscapes, and most of all, mineral springs. Of these, Baden-Baden enjoyed the most extensive coverage, but many pages were devoted to smaller watering places, such as Sulzbach and Rippoldsau, which drew only a handful of visitors at this time. For each, the *Handbuch* presented historical, geographical, and practical information, such as hotel facilities and the like, but then devoted a substantial segment to discussion of the therapeutic efficacy of their mineral springs and the opportunities available for their use. In this respect as well, the most space was devoted to Baden-Baden; smaller towns, the

---

[29] Eugen Guinot, *Ein Sommer in Baden-Baden*. (Leipzig: J.J. Weber, 1858), 189. This guide was evidently rather popular, appearing in German, French and English editions.

[30] H. Schreiber, *Handbuch für Eisenbahn-Reisende durch das Grossherzogthum Baden, nebst den Reiserouten durch das Neckarthal, über den Schwarzwald und nach den Seegegenden* (Karlsruhe, Chr. Fr. Müller'sche Hofbuchhandlung, 1846).

author remarked with regret, lacked the infrastructure to allow fuller exploitation of their springs.

Smaller spas also lacked the glamour and glitz of Baden-Baden, and drew a modest, mostly local clientele. The larger spas offered a full range of attractions, and consequently, attracted a diverse public. Alongside nobles and bourgeois notables, who tended to stay in expensive first-class luxury hotels, one also found a significant number of patrons similar to those found in smaller spas, who predominated in more modest hotels in Baden-Baden and Wiesbaden, for instance small merchants, school teachers and lower-grade civil servants.[31] In provincial spa towns, as Lewald remarked, "the springs dominate, and as a consequence, their effects push all else aside … Those uninterested, that is, the healthy, therefore stay away, and the entertainments that such a spa offers are devised for the sick and convalescent."[32] At the same time, he referred to Baden-Baden as "a sort of occidental Mecca, to which all of the faithful must undertake the pilgrimage once in their lifetime. And among these faithful there are many to be counted, who believe in the infallibility of the Martingale, as well as those who believe in the certitude of the medical arts and science."[33] It is reasonable to conclude, then, that although the glamour of spas like Baden-Baden and Wiesbaden attracted a number of healthy, pleasure-seeking individuals not in the least interested in curing, so too, did they attract significant numbers of travelers seeking a cure of their ailments. Entertainment, gambling and leisure were the salient features of the grand spas in this period, yet they did not overwhelm the medicinal use of the waters. Visitors came not only to relax and be amused, or to try their luck, but also to take the waters.

Statistics kept by the spa administration in Baden-Baden support this conclusion. As early as 1829, the spa committee sought to gather information regarding not only the number of guests housed in each bathing establishment but also the number of baths of various types they administered. Much to the chagrin of the leading *Badearzt,* who had been charged with gathering the data, the reports remained incomplete and unreliable throughout the 1830s and 1840s, possibly because competitive-minded proprietors were reluctant to disclose information. By midcentury, however, their compliance had improved, and starting in 1853, reliable reports were compiled.[34]

---

[31] Bitz, *Badewesen in Südwestdeutschland*, 316.
[32] August Lewald, "Bilder aus Baden-Baden," 962.
[33] August Lewald, "Bilder aus Baden-Baden," 962.
[34] GLAKa 195/995, "Die Badanstalten zu Baden, insbesondere gesundheitliche Reglement für dieselben, Zusammenstellungen über die Zahl und Art der

As the number of guests increased, so too did the number of medicinal baths given. In 1856, for example, 67,754 baths of various kinds were given in seventeen different establishments. Over 21,000 or nearly one third of all baths, were given in the two finest, and most expensive, hotels in town, the *Badischer Hof* and the *Darmstädter Hof*. At the other end of the spectrum, just over one sixth were administered in the charitable bath for the poor (*Armenbad*) and the least expensive hotel in town, the *Baldreit*. The largest number, over 30,000, were taken by persons presumably of moderate, yet respectable means staying in the mid-range establishments.[35]

Precisely how many guests made use of the baths is difficult to determine, but evidence suggests that the number was significant. The Wiesbaden *Badearzt* Gustav Heinrich Richter estimated in 1841, that 47% of all visitors were proper *Kurgäste*, staying for a cure.[36] This may well be an exaggeration made by a promotion-minded physician seeking to advance his practice. Doctors in the *Armenbad*, for which better records are available, generally prescribed two baths a week during a curative regimen of three weeks, supported by drinking mineral water, diet, and exercise. At an average of nearly 1.5 baths per person, and if a prescription during a cure was for three baths a week, a reasonable conclusion is that at least one in four visitors made regular use of the baths for treatment, which would not include those simply taking the popular drinking cure. This drinking cure was clearly medicinal and not an amusement. Aside from being prescribed by physicians, most spa water was (and is) notoriously foul in both taste and smell, as a visit to Baden-Baden today can confirm. Consequently, the number of visitors who were at the spa for curative purposes was likely one in three or more.

The physical development of the spa also lends support to this conclusion. The construction of new facilities in nearly all spas substantiates greater demand and Guinot's anecdotal evidence that curing remained an important element of the major spas. Baden-Baden, for example, met the demands of an expanding number of bourgeois visitors with the construction of a new, imposing neoclassical *Trinkhalle* adorned with representative nationalistic frescos in 1850 –evidently chosen by the authorities in Karlsruhe to adopt, reflect, and possibly co-opt the nationalist sentiments expressed in 1848. A replacement for the 1820s era

---

verabreichten Bäder. (BAKom) 1853-1862." Summary reports are available in this file for the years 1853-59.

[35] GLAKa 195/995, "Zusammenstellung der im Jahr 1856 abgegebenen Bäder."

[36] Gustav Heinrich Richter, *Kur- und Lebensregeln für Wiesbaden's Brunnengäste*. (Düsseldorf: J.H.C. Schreiner, 1842), vii.

steam bath was constructed in 1846-1851, but not without some controversy. Many physicians felt that the old facility was sufficient, and that a new one based on Russian-style steam baths was not necessary. Karl Frech, a medical doctor who owned and operated the mid-rank Hotel *Hirsch* that offered a small private Russian steam bath after 1841, contended that it was the demand of the curing public more than his colleagues that gave the administration impetus to approve the new construction.[37]

Direct testimony regarding the use of these facilities in this period, unfortunately, is as scarce as for he earlier era, although personal letters and memoirs can cast some light on what people actually did in the spas. Social interaction and amusement of course remained, as ever, prominent, but curing was far from absent. Scant attention is paid in these sources to the "mundane" aspects of a spa-visit, and consequently one finds little in the way of discussions of specific therapies or cures. Letter-writers preferred to highlight the aspects of their visit that were interesting to them, such as who they may have met, an exciting excursion, and so forth. This is not to say, however, that these did not play an important role in the experience. With such sources, the historian must read carefully and cautiously to find what was then universally assumed –spa visit often included consulting a physician and taking a cure.

The renowned pathologist Rudolf Virchow, a man certainly well-versed in the trends of medical treatment, described several times in letters to his father how the spas were used for curative purposes. He wrote of a "sick friend … who was in Bad Soden bei Frankfurt for her health" in 1853,[38] and in 1856 how his father-in-law spent several weeks in Wiesbaden for treatment of an orthopedic ailment.[39] Otto von Bismarck spent substantial periods of time in the grand spas, occupied with the work of politics and diplomacy. Despite his constant activity, however, he found time to take the waters. In 1859, following a leg injury in Russia that was exacerbated by the "ignorance and impudence of the medical swindler" -- a Russian physician who had treated him. Bismarck next consulted Piragov, the famous Russian surgeon and inventor of the plaster cast, who

---

[37] Carl Frech, *Die Russischen Thermaldampfbader in Baden-Baden*, (Lahr: Verlag von M. Schauenberg & C., 1862), 9-11.

[38] Rudolf Virchow, *Sämtliche Werke*, Christian Andree, ed. Band 59, Abteilung IV: Briefwechsel mit den Eltern 1839-1864, zum ersten Mal vollständig in historisch-kritischer Edition, (Berlin, Vienna: Blackwell Wissenschafts-Verlag, 2001), 194

[39] Virchow, *Sämtliche Werke*, Christian Andree, ed. Band 59, Abteilung IV, 249–252.

suggested amputation. Instead, "in order to find help from German doctors" he returned home and was finally healed "by the baths of Nauheim," a smaller spa in Nassau.[40] Nor was this an isolated incident: in letters to his wife from 1863 and 1864, Bismarck told how in the Austrian spa Bad Gastein he took "twenty-one or twenty-two baths in twenty-six days."[41]

Bismarck, a notorious hypochondriac, habitually took baths when in a spa town, apparently complying with the regimen prescribed by a physician. Taking the waters, however, did not necessarily translate into automatic trust in physicians. This was not peculiar to Bismarck, but was fairly common at midcentury. An 1854 article in the *Morgenblatt* makes this clear:

> There is an odd play around the doctors gathered at the spring, who hold their audiences there, and the hardly edified public watches and listens. These people cannot really heal, it is not in their power, they are only the agents of those doctors who have sent their patients here, they are only the momentary executive authority, that extracts a small levy, by which they do quite well.[42]

Bismarck, then was not alone in his reluctance to put too much faith in the authority of spa physicians. Despite his successful treatment in 1859, he remained suspicious, occasionally contemptuous, of doctors, and indeed of mineral waters, writing to his ill wife in 1864, that he was "strongly inclined to look for the blame [for her illness] among doctors, mineral water and medications,"[43] and later that "grapes help more than poison from the pharmacy." Yet in a twist typical for many spa patrons of the middle and upper echelons of society, Bismarck was clearly ambivalent, cherishing his skepticism but still clinging to some hope that physicians and their springs could in fact heal. Physicians and spa enthusiasts could always point to cases in which therapy was apparently successful, and this no doubt exerted an influence. In a later letter from Baden bei Wien, for example, Bismarck wrote his wife how he felt encouraged from many

---

[40] Otto Fürst von Bismarck, *Gedanken und Erinnerungen*. Neue Ausgabe. Stuttgart and Berlin: J.G. Cotta'sche Buchhandlung Nachfolger, 1921, 1: 269.

[41] Letter from Bismarck to his wife, August 14 1863, in *Fürst Bismarcks Briefe an seine Braut und Gattin,* Fürst Herert Bismarck, ed. (Stuttgart: J.G. Cotta'sche Buchhandlung Nachfolger, 1900), 528.

[42] "Korrespondenz-Nachrichten. Marienbad, Juli. Ursprung des Bades–Saison," *Morgenblatt für gebildete Leser* 33 (August 13, 1854), 784.

[43] Letter from Bismarck to his wife, September 5, 1864, in Bismarck, *Briefe an seine Braut und Gattin,* 547.

sides to take the bathing cure, observing how one companion "felt like a new man after only three baths."[44]

Bismarck was no ordinary middle-class spa patron, by any stretch of the imagination. His letters, however, are more forthcoming about medicine and the spa than those of many middle-class patrons. Virchow's letters to his father, stating the facts but remaining silent on details of treatments or of his feelings about them are typical, given that nineteenth-century letter-writers tended to be reticent regarding such issues. Personal testimonials, then, are a source problem that other historians working on the nineteenth century health spa have also encountered, especially in the German case.[45] Americans taking a cure in Saratoga Springs were far less circumspect about their experiences, writing directly about the laxative effect of large doses of spring water.[46] Where American guidebooks consisted in large part of patient testimonials, discreet yet direct, German guides rested more on physicians' assertions of the salutary properties of the cure. Published works, too, respected the boundaries of propriety. Heinrich Laube, for instance, made only a veiled reference to the purgative properties of spring water in describing how an attendant in a *Trinkhalle* smiled inwardly when he bought a sheet of fine grade paper with the intent of securing some reading material, for "the paper was not intended for such common purposes."[47]

Given the inhibition of German authors to address intimate and delicate issues directly, their testimony is only of limited usefulness in understanding the views of spa patrons toward physicians and the practice of medicine. Humor and satire, on the other hand, can often speak to issues that otherwise remain unaddressed in more polite forms of discourse. *Hans-Jörgels Badereise*, part of an ongoing popular weekly series published in Vienna for over forty years, was written in letter-form in an Austrian country dialect, rife with misspellings.[48] Using the voice of a

---

[44] Letter from Bismarck to his wife, October 3, 1864, *Briefe an seine Braut und Gattin*, 549.

[45] Personal correspondence between the author and Heikki Lempa, June 6, 2000.

[46] Thomas A. Chambers, *Drinking the Waters. Creating an American Leisure Class at Nineteenth-Century Mineral Springs* (Washington and London: Smithsonian Institution Press, 2002), 68

[47] Heinrich Laube, "Marienbad," in *Heinrich Laube, Reise durch das Biedermeier*, 131.

[48] The full title of the series, *Komische Briefe des Hans-Jörgel von Gumpoldskirchen an seinen Schwager Maxel in Feselau,* appeared weekly from 1837-1879. The version referenced in this work is not a periodical, but rather a bound edition, *Hans-Jörgels Badereise*, Vols. 1 & 2 (Vienna: Bauer und Dirnböck, 1842). No author is given in the volume itself, but the catolog reference at the

simple country bumpkin talking to his relatives back home, the author could hide behind the uncouth provincial while describing matters respectable people were expected to avoid. A literal illustration of this point is found on the title page, which included a full-color illustration of guests standing around the mineral spring, and showed a middle-class man making an urgent dash for the nearest privy, clutching his abdomen with an unmistakably distressed mien.

Under the cover of satire, then, the author could be far more forthcoming than the reputable Heinrich Laube. *Hans-Jörgels Badereise*, adorned with the subtitle of an "indispensable handbook for everyone who does not wish to make the tour, but who still wants to know what one eats, drinks, thinks and says in other places, and what one can see and hear there,"[49] was evidently intended for the entertainment of armchair travelers or, likely, given its pocket-sized format and inexpensive paper, for those actually making the trip. In the work, the author mockingly tells of the journey of a rural naïf, Hans-Jörgel, to the spas of Karlsbad and Franzensbad in Bohemia to seek treatment for his injured foot and, in a clear pun on antiquated Galenic medicine, his injured humor. First, the protagonist consulted several physicians, each prescribing a different treatment or none at all. After much vexation with the medical community, he at last took the advice of a stranger and decided to try the mud baths in Franzensbad.

The fictional *Badereise* is filled with a colorful cast of characters, always seen through the supposedly innocent eyes of the eponymous traveler and given an ironic twist by the author. These figures represented a cross-section of the spa world, ranging from a charlatan masquerading as a professor, most interested in seducing Hans-Jörgel's traveling companion, a middle-aged female sauerkraut maker traveling on a doctor's orders, musicians and artists, including the above mentioned Heinrich Laube, to a count and countess from Hanover, who to Hans-Jörgel's surprise, were "really sweet people, and have learned more than how many branches their family tree has or how many cows they have standing in the stall."[50]

The most relevant remarks for this study, however, are those regarding medicine, curing, and doctors, even though these subjects were also treated with much good-humored irony. In the pages of *Hans-Jörgels Badereise*, physicians appear befuddled, if well-intended healers. In the

---

Staatsbibliothek Preussischer Kulturbesitz zu Berlin (Yb 17969) lists the author as Johann Baptist Weis.

[49] *Hans-Jörgels Badereise*, 1:1.

[50] *Hans-Jörgels Badereise,* 2: 130.

narrator's words, "[d]octors, when they don't know what to do with their patients, send them to a spa," because "what no medicine could ever heal and can't heal, a mineral spring should cure."[51] Hans-Jörgel encounters patients of all kinds, with a full spectrum of symptoms and expectations:

> What kind of demands people make of such a spring is unbelievable. If one has a red nose, a real schnoz, then he thinks all he has to do is drink mineral water and it will shrink. Another one is a little heavy-set, and has to get thin again, if he takes the cure; the skinny ones hope to get fat again; one has too much blood, another has too little; one has excited, the other dulled nerves; one has something wrong with his head, the other in his stomach. One has a pressure on the right side, the other feels a pinch on the left.
>
> [Was d'Leut für Anforderungen an so ein Brunn machen, dös sollt man nit glaubn. Hat Einer eine rothe Nasen, so ein rechten Schmecker, so glaubt er, er darf nur Mineralwasser trinken, und sie wird z'sammenfalln. Ein Zweiter is ein Bisserl stark beleibt, der muß wieder mager werdn, wann er die Kur braucht; die Magern hoffen wieder, daß's fett werden; Einer hat z'viel Blut, der And're hat z'wenig; Einer hat aufg'regte, der And're abg'süannte Nerven; Einem fehlts im Kopf, dem Andern im Magn; Einen druckts rehts, den Andern zwickt's links [all *sic*].[52]

Another episode lampooned warnings about the supposedly irresponsible use of the waters without scrupulously following a physician's expert advice. At the spring, the only distraction from the tales of amazing cures told by patients was the account of a Russian who perished after misunderstanding his doctor's instructions, and drank far too much of the wondrous tonic. This, for Hans-Jörgel, proved "in what senseless and dumb ways some people lose their lives, who don't ask a doctor for advice, but rather take the cure on their own."[53]

Hans-Jörgels Badereise was not, however, totally skeptical about the salubrious effects of a spa visit. The narrator concedes that most people left the spa healthier than when they arrived, owing to a combination of the waters and their therapeutic use, as well as diet and exercise in the fresh air. Hans-Jörgel himself finds relief from his affliction in the mud baths. As a whole, this midcentury portrayal of hapless, feuding doctors was far less acerbic, far more forgiving, than Jean-Paul's rendering in the

---

[51] *Hans-Jörgels Badereise,* 2: 123.
[52] *Hans-Jörgels Badereise*, 2: 122-123. The original of this excerpt is cited as well in order to give a sense of the character of the prose and style.
[53] *Hans-Jörgels Badereise*, 2: 93.

first decade of the century, which pilloried physicians as macabre merchants of death in league with the devil (see Chapter Three) The contrast suggests that by midcentury people more readily took the doctor's advice in order to seek relief from their maladies, even if they had some reservations about its efficacy. Underneath the satire of *Hans-Jörgels Badereise*, one can discern an ambivalence about physicians and their remedies similar to Bismarck's. Resentment of the doctors' professional omniscience in the face of indisputable evidence pointing to the limitations to their ability to heal coexisted with a hopeful resignation that there was something to it, after all. Although they viewed the doctor's prescription with suspicion, they could also observe that the waters often did seem to provide relief, particularly from chronic ailments.

This was clearly a rational compromise on the part of spa-goers, especially in this period when the inefficacy of most treatments was obvious enough to spark a movement within academic medicine of "therapeutic nihilism," which entailed abstinence from therapy altogether because of an extremely limited ability to offer effective and scientifically grounded treatment.[54] In the face of such narrow options, taking the waters as a cure, as in the first decades of the century, gave the infirm a sense of doing something that contributed to their recovery, or that was at least a useful palliative, and others a sense of maintaining their health.

A sufficient number of guests availed themselves of the waters and sought medical counsel that by midcentury, some spa physicians complained of the lack of sufficient space to see all their patients.[55] In large part, these continued to practice medicine as they had for years. Yet herein lay a problem. In the decades when curing at the spa was overshadowed by the glitz of light-hearted distractions, spa medicine stagnated in Romantic natural philosophy and the notion of the "*Brunnengeist*," often referred to as electricity. Basking in the warm glow of gulden and a steady flow of patients to the spas, perhaps out of conviction, perhaps out of complacency, the practice of spa medicine had by the 1830s grown stagnant, just as it faced a challenge from a new method of hydrotherapy devised by a layman, Vincenz Priessnitz.

Priessnitz was seen by many nearly as a prophet of a new form of therapy using cold water rather than the thermal mineral water found in the

---

[54] Wolfgang U. Eckhart, *Geschichte der Medizin*, 3rd revised edition. (Berlin: Springer Verlag, 1998), 262.

[55] Joachim Moerchel, *Die Nassauischen Badeärzte in ihrer wissenschaftlichen und praktischen Tätigkeit 1816-1866*, European University Papers Series VII, Health Sciences-Division B History of Medicine, Vol. 1 (Frankfurt am Main: Peter Lang, 1977), 237.

grand spas. Physicians generally reviled the medicinal use of ordinary water, especially by laypersons or practitioners who, as K.A. Zwierlein hotly argued at the beginning of the nineteenth century, would likely do more harm than good. Many among the curing public did not share his view, and by the beginning of the third decade of the nineteenth century turned to Priessnitz at his establishment in the small Silesian town of Gräfenberg.

Priessnitz was exactly what spa doctors had most scorned and feared: a man with no formal medical training who developed and applied a hydrotherapeutic course of therapy that patients–customers–found at least as effective of those of medical doctors. A simple country man without any formal education, Priessnitz became interested in cold-water therapy after observing how local peasants wrapped their horses' and cows' injuries in cloths soaked in cold water. After conducting experiments on himself, drawing on traditions of Silesian folk medicine, Priessnitz began to treat others in the same fashion. By 1826, his reputation spreading, people began to travel to Gräfenberg to undergo his treatment. In 1831 the farmer turned *Wasserdoktor* received official permission from the Austrian government to receive and treat patients in his cold-water therapy establishment.[56]

Inspired by the growing number of patients seeking out his assistance for a host of ailments, Priessnitz developed an ever-wider range of therapies. His 1847 *Familien Wasserbuch* reveals a combination of over fifty hydrotherapeutic applications to treat both chronic and acute illnesses.[57] Patients were expected to submit to a Spartan regimen that in ways echoed the daily routine that doctors prescribed for patients in the grand spas, with critical differences, however, that resulted in a much different environment in Gräfenberg than in the thermal bath towns. First, Priessnitz' operation stood alone in the locale, facing no competition from rival therapists or guest facilities. This allowed Priessnitz to maintain significant control. His authority was bolstered by the fact that the only persons accepted in Gräfenberg were those willing to comply with his therapeutic regime. Although a spa-like social scene did emerge in Gräfenberg, which by 1840 did have a modest *Kurhaus* (significantly

[56] Horst Prignitz, *Wasserkur und Badelust: Eine Badereise in die Vergangenheit* (Leipzig: Koehler & Amelang, 1986), 179.

[57] For a more detailed discussion of Priessnitz' therapeutic regimens, see J. Rohde, "In Vergessenheit geratene Erkenntnisse über Priessnitz aus dem unbekannt gebliebenen Vinzenz Priessnitz'schen Familien-Wasserbuch von 1847," *Forschende Komplementärmedizin und Klassische Naturheilkunde* 9 (2002): 85-98.

without a casino) and comfortable lodging, an atmosphere of serious curing was maintained such that spa physicians could only dream of.

In Gräfenberg, patients rose at four in the morning to begin their treatment by being tightly wrapped in damp cloths and covered with a woolen blanket to sit for several hours of sweating before enduring a shocking cold immersion and several more hours walking in the woods drinking cold water. Only then was a sparse breakfast of milk and bread served. This meager fare was followed again by more cold water, more exercise, another simple meal, and again walks in the forest.[58] A variant drinking cure required imbibing up to thirty glasses daily, and an icy shower completely nude beneath a waterfall in the forest.[59] Conversation and sociability were to be confined to meal times, and the amusements of the watering places were kept strictly in check, restricted to dancing on Sundays.[60] Smoking, alcohol, use of spices, and a range of other unhealthy habits were strictly prohibited.[61] In Gräfenberg, rigorous curing stood unassailably in the center of the entire experience.

This rigor was evidently attractive. The number of guests taking Priessnitz' cure annually rose steadily, from 200 in 1833 to 2,000 in 1840. The social composition of the visitors changed as well, from local artisans and farmers in the 1820s, to wealthy middle-class and noble patrons from across all German lands and abroad.[62] Gräfenberg drew its share of notables as well, with such figures in its guest registry as Nikolai Gogol, Frederic Chopin, and Prince Gorchakov.[63] In this sense, the small Silesian town proved the equal of the grand spas, assuming its place on the circuit of water curing for the modest and the prominent alike.

---

[58] Sigfried Giedion, *Geschichte des Bades* (Hamburg: Europäische Verlagsanstalt, 1998), 42.

[59] Prignitz, *Wasserkur und Badelust*, 180.

[60] Heinz Sponsel, *Der Heilkräfte der Natur*, cited in Gernot von Hahn, Hans-Kaspar von Schönfels, *Wunderbares Wasser. Von der heilsamen Kraft der Brunnen und Bäder*, 2nd edition (Aarau, Stuttgart: AT Verlag, 1986), 94.

[61] Prignitz, *Wasserkur und Badelust*, 189.

[62] Prignitz, *Wasserkur und Badelust*, 190. See also Christian Andree, "Einleitung" to Ernst von Held-Ritt, *Prißnitz auf Gräfenberg oder treue Darstellung seines Heilverfahrens mit kaltem Wasser: ein Handbuch für alle, welche Gräfenberg besuchen, und der Wasserkur dort oder in die Heimath brauchen wollen so wie für jene, welche dort Heilung fanden / mit einer Einleitung. zur Geschichte der Hydrotherapie und der Biographie von Prießnitz sowie mit Erläuterungen und Anmerkungen. hrsg. von Christian Andree.* Expanded second edition of the original, Mörschner u. Jasper, Wien, 1837 (Würzburg: Berstadtverlag Korn, 1988), 11.

[63] Hahn and Schönfels, *Wunderbares Wasser*, 94.

It was likely a combination of Priessnitz' personal charisma with his apparent success as a healer that drew followers. Experience with his establishment was able to win the admiration of educated individuals who initially had been skeptical of the Silesian farmer. One such convert was a gymnasium professor from Ansbach in Bavaria, Eucharius Ferdinand Christian Oertel, who in 1830 had denounced Priessnitz as "yet another water doctor," by 1834 had published a tract calling on all governments in Germany to found therapeutic establishments on Priessnitz' model, and became one of the main promoters of Priessnitz' method in Germany.[64] Nor was Oertel alone in his praise for Priessnitz and his methods, as the many works published in this period testify.[65]

Priessnitz' success drew the attention of the medical establishment as well, both in the form of positive interest and alarm from physicians suspicious of this lay upstart. In 1829 Priessnitz was confronted with accusations of quackery and of using magic. He was absolved of these charges after an investigation conducted by Ludwig Freiherr von Türkheim, who found that Priessnitz' therapies "proved in many respects to be salutary" and prohibition difficult and perhaps counterproductive, as Gräfenberg was popular among Viennese society.[66] Others came to observe and learn, such as a the military surgeon R.J. Scoutetten, who was sent by the French government in 1843.[67] This interest inspired imitation as well, and by 1850, water-cure establishments using Priessnitz' methods had sprung up not only across Central Europe, but in Ireland and the United States.

While many in the medical establishment remained highly skeptical of the "water doctor" and his methods, others became followers. One well-documented case is the Swabian surgeon, Johann Bernhard Zipperlen. The son of a military surgeon, Zipperlen studied surgery in Vienna and Würzburg, earning the title of medical doctor before coming to Gräfenberg

---

[64] Andree, "Einleitung," 19.

[65] Eucharius Ferdinand Christian Oertel, *Vincenz Priessnitz oder ein Aufruf an alle Staatsregierungen Deutschlands zur Einrichtung von Wasserheilanstalten*. 1834, cited in Prignitz, *Wasserkur und Badelust*, 179. See also for example Ernst von Held-Ritt, *Prißnitz auf Gräfenberg* or Leopold von der Decken-Himmelreich, *Priessnitz und die Wasserkur: Aertze und Allopathie wissenschaftlich konfrontirt* (Breslau: 1845).

[66] Prignitz, pp. 153-154. Türkheim was a physician and jurist, Chancellor of the University of Vienna in 1817 and 1829, and vice-director of the medical-surgical college in Vienna. See *AEIOU, Das Kulturinformationssystem des Bundesministerium für Bildung, Wissenschaft und Kultur* [Austria], at http://www.aeiou.at/aeiou.encyclop.t/t950672.htm, accessed July 14, 2004.

[67] Giedion, *Geschichte des Bades*, 40.

in 1838 to learn from Priessnitz. He then pursued a career as a *Badearzt* in the smaller spa towns of Herrenalb and Teinach from 1849 until his retirement in 1854. Priessnitz' influence is evident in Zipperlen's 1844 *Hülfsbüchlein für Gesundheitslehre für alle Stände*, a guide for persons of all stations in life on the home use of cold-water therapy according to Priessnitz' teachings.[68]

The *Hülfsbüchlein* resembles in some ways the guides to the grand spas, yet is significantly divergent in spirit. Drawing on authorities like Goethe's physician, the highly-esteemed Christoph Wilhelm Hufeland, the Swabian surgeon offered clear, explicit advice on the proper and safe way to use water for the maintenance of health and the treatment of disease, and warned the reader of the dangers of misuse. Like Priessnitz, Zipperlen strongly emphasized the importance of personal bathing, the consumption of clean fresh water and exercise in fresh air for health.

Zipperlen, much like the authors of medical guidebooks to the grand spas, was confident of his expertise and the danger that readers would face by flaunting his advice. At the same time, and in marked contrast to the spa doctors, he entrusted the educated lay reader with responsibility for his or her own health. The stated purpose of the volume was to enable readers to safely use water therapeutically at home. The authors of conventional guides, on the other hand, provided readers with partial information, but admonished again and again never to attempt any cure without the careful direction of an expert physician, ideally, one could presume, the author himself.

Whatever his own motivation, Zipperlen's attitude toward self-treatment evidenced in his *Hülfsbüchlein* distinguished him from the mainstream of spa medicine in that he clearly represented an alternative to the conventional medicine of the time. This was not lost upon the cohort of spa physicians. Cold-water therapies presented a two-fold danger to them. First, obviously enough, Gräfenberg and similar establishments threatened to draw away their most lucrative clientele, the sick seeking medical help and possibly those who were well, but worried about their health. Those seeking amusement would not be too likely to visit Gräfenberg, but these would not provide as much business as the truly ill for a spa physician's practice. Cold-water therapy threatened to draw away the base of paying

---

[68] Johann Bernhard Zipperlen, *Hülfsbüchlein für Gesundheitslehre für alle Stände. Eine gemeinnützige Anleitung zum wirksamen Gebrauch des kalten Wassers* (Stuttgart: Verlag der J.F. Steintopf'schen Buchhandlung, 1844). A handwritten copy of Zipperlen's obituary in the *Stuttgarter Zeitung* was written on the inside cover the copy of the book in the University of Tübingen library (call number JK 149), evidently by a descendant who donated the book to the university's collection.

patients –a physician's nightmare to be sure. Worse, however, was that a layman had devised a popular method for water therapy. This undermined the spa doctor's long campaign to have his authority and knowledge recognized. Works like Zipperlen's only exacerbated the damage already done by the Silesian country remedy, at once legitimizing it with the seal of approval of someone from the profession and dangerously proposing that intelligent people could apply it at home on their own.

Thus the practices of a layman who presented a viable alternative therapy spread beyond his own establishment, even to some physicians. The popularity of Gräfenberg declined rapidly after the healer's death in 1851, leaving behind an association between cold-water therapy as an alternative to academic medicine. Nevertheless, physicians in the large spas were not tempted to imitate the Silesian success. They dreaded being perceived as practitioners of an alternative medicine. Rather, they clung desperately to the desire to be seen as part of the mainstream academic establishment.

The popularity of Priessnitz' cold-water therapy, together with the spreading view that entertainment took precedence at places like Baden-Baden, combined to erode the large spas' reputation as places of serious curing. The threat, however, did not arise solely from forces beyond the spa physicians' control. Their science had also come under attack. In growing measure, hydrotherapy had ceased to be counted among "the most respected branches of medicine." As the study of medicine advanced in the 1830s, 40s and 50s, spa doctors lagged behind.[69] The water healers' self-promotion, self-satisfaction, and obstinacy only contributed to their problems.

Guides from Baden-Baden, Wiesbaden, and Ems continued to insist on the authoritative position of the physician. So, for example, the Wiesbaden spa physician Gustav Heinrich Richter cautioned in his 1842 guide, *Kur- und Lebensregeln für Wiesbaden's Brunnengäste* [sic],[70] that the "spa guest ... can only halfway or very incompletely understand its content."[71] He nonetheless provided general rules to promote both the health of

[69] Johannes Steudel, "Geschichte der Bäder- und Klimaheilkunde," in *Handbuch der Bäder- und Klimaheilkunde*, Walther Amelung and Arrien Evers, eds. (Stuttgart, Schattauer-Verlag, 1962), 16.
[70] Gustav Heinrich Richter, *Kur- und Lebensregeln für Wiesbaden's Brunnengäste* (Düsseldorf: Verlag von J.H.C. Schreiner, 1842). Richter, a doctor of medicine and surgery practiced as a spa physican in Wiesbaden, and gave as additional qualifications–typically for this type of guide–membership in twelve associations for medicine and culture across Germany.
[71] Richter, *Kur- und Lebensregeln*, v.

patients, and one might presume more importantly, to protect the reputation of his spa by ensuring that visitors acted responsibly, that is, by following doctors' orders. In the chapter on general rules for the cure, Richter warned readers how a little knowledge was a dangerous thing. He wrote sternly:

> It is not a rare occurrence that patients dare to use the healing springs here at their own discretion without the advice of any physician, in part because they believe that nothing more is necessary for the cure than to drink a certain number of glasses from the spring daily and to take a bath, without sensing the effect of this powerful treatment, sometimes because they believe to have acquired medical knowledge through reading popular medical guides, sometimes, however, as is unfortunately more often the case, because they come equipped with instructions from their physician at home for using the mineral springs.[72]

Even more dangerous, in Richter's view, was that patients shared their experiences with each other, which resulted in the uncomfortable situation that "nowhere is medical quackery more prevalent than in a spa."[73]

The only way to avoid the dangers of quackery, Richter argued, was to seek advice from a specialist at the spa, like himself, who was expert in the effects of the waters, which could be unpredictable. On the surface, these admonitions to patients are strikingly similar to those raised in guides earlier in the century, as discussed in the previous chapter: one should never, under any circumstances, take the waters without proper medical attention. But the tone evinced in Richter's guide had changed, becoming more strident, attempting to keep pace with the mounting and multiple threats to the spa doctor's authority.

What constituted proper medical attention had also changed by the 1840s. Richter's guide suggests two related developments. More patients were in fact coming to the spa after having consulted a physician, as both *Hans-Jörgels Badereise* and Bismarck's letters suggest. This, however, was no longer regarded as adequate preparation, as "the specific prescriptions of one's home physician will not help him [i.e., a patient] at all."[74] Essential for the success of a cure, then, was seeking not just medical counsel, but that of an expert in the field of water cures, foreshadowing the development of greater specialization in medicine. This hint at specialization is still only tentative. Medical guidebooks such as

---

[72] Richter, *Kur- und Lebensregeln*, 43-44.
[73] Richter, *Kur- und Lebensregeln*, 44.
[74] Richter, *Kur- und Lebensregeln*, 45.

Richter's, just as earlier in the century, at once cautioned patients about the dangers of applying limited knowledge and paradoxically still supplied them with that very knowledge. It was an uneasy balance, evidently driven by the demand for such information more than any faith in people being able to use it correctly. It was likely a concession to the reality that a good number of cure-seekers did not bother consulting an expert in the spa. Richter, perhaps, hoped that dazzling readers with his expertise in print, and frightening them with threats of the mortal danger posed by either treating themselves or following inexpert prescriptions, would draw patients to his practice.

The bold claims of the extraordinary rewards of the "proper" use of the waters continued unabated into midcentury and beyond. Guidebooks of all sorts presented the same promises and claims: when properly applied by an expert physician, the waters could cure almost anything. The list of maladies which they could purportedly remedy is astonishing. One finds that most springs had the power to heal not only chronic illnesses such as gout and rheumatism, but anemia, inflammations, broken bones, diseases of the liver, pancreas, kidneys, and gastrointestinal tract; they were reported useful for treating dermatological conditions, nervous disorders, hypochondria, and deafness, as well as syphilis and female infertility.[75] Just how believable these claims were to nineteenth-century readers is impossible to determine, but, given the repetitiveness and extravagance of the claims, it seems fair to assume that they met with a fair amount of healthy skepticism.

Even what may have appeared to be more responsible behavior on the part of some physicians may not have been entirely disinterested. Some spa doctors distanced themselves from panacea claims, and stressed in their works that certain waters were suitable only for particular maladies. There are cases in which practitioners referred patients to other spas where their ills could be more suitably treated. But frequently these referrals would be to another spa within the same territory, such as from Wiesbaden to Ems, both in Nassau and under the same state administration. Since

[75] Many medical guides of the time make similar claims, either for the waters of the spa the author was promoting, or for a combination of its waters combined with artificial Karlsbad water (also available there, of course). See for example, [first name not given] Kramer, *Ueber die Eigenschaften, Wirkungen und den zweckmäßigen Gebrauch der warmen Mineralquelle, so wie der natürlichen Stahlbäder zu Baden im Großherzogthume...* (Karlsruhe und Baden, Marx'sche Buchhandlung, 1830), [first name not given] Halffter, *Die See-Bade-Anstalten zu Zoppot bei Danzig in ihrem gegenwärtigen Zustande* (Danzig: Wedel'sche Hofbuchdruckerei, 1842).

many of the more reputable practitioners were state officials, they were in fact promoting another branch of the same enterprise.[76]

However, there were indeed some conscientious spa physicians who behaved responsibly. They sensed a threat to their professional credibility posed by excessive claims of near miraculous cures, noting that the promotional efforts of irresponsible colleagues undermined the standing of the entire field of spa medicine. Even so, these practitioners also faced criticism from the medical world outside the spa for their lack of scientific discipline. An exchange in the pages of the *Balneologische Zeitung*, a weekly journal dedicated to improving the scientific footing of the discipline, illustrates this point clearly. A reader, one Dr. Bolle in Paderborn, offered severe criticism in a letter responding to an article which had praised the healing properties of the waters in two small spas. He lambasted the author for offering vague, unfounded claims of how "the waters improve the blood after all," without any clear description of how, specifically, this occurs. He continued, "[this] has to change, if anything is to come of balneology–because until now it has been nothing other than a bright mishmash of unripe, half-observations, which are clouded by unproven hypotheses and rendered useless to such an extent that it is 'a crying shame." He concluded that the only hope for any future for the discipline is through proper scientific experimentation.[77] Such harsh criticism could not go unchallenged. The author, the *Brunnenarzt* Schnackenberg, replied in clear terms. The article, he claimed, was only a preliminary report; more could be found in a descriptive monograph. He then responded defensively with his own series of questions, but conceded that ultimately, the findings rested on years of observations in clinical practice.[78]

Herein lay the crux of the issue. As discussed in the previous chapter, spa medicine in the early decades of the century had been empirically based, ascribing much to the inexplicable properties of the waters. This tendency continued into subsequent decades. The face of medicine was changing, however, to demand a more scientific, experimentally verifiable approach. The figure who perhaps most strongly represented this new

---

[76] See Joachim Moerchel, *Die Nassauischen Badeärzte*.

[77] "Kritik, Hofgeismar und Elster betreffend. Briefliche Mittheilung and die Redaction von Dr. Bolle in Paderborn," *Balneologische Zeitung. Correspondenzblatt der deutschen Gesellschaft für Hydrologie* 1, no. 9 (April 23, 1855): 175-176.

[78] "Zur Kritik des Herrn Dr. Bolle über die Heilwirkungen und Nachrichten von den Kurorten Hofgeismar und Elster. Von Dr. Schackenberg, Brunnenarzt zu Hofgeismar." *Balneologische Zeitung. Correspondenzblatt der deutschen Gesellschaft für Hydrologie* 1, no. 9 (April 23, 1855): 176-180.

direction in German academic medicine was the pathologist Rudolf Virchow. Virchow's approach to medicine, in which cellular pathology played a central role, largely helped establish the methodological standards of modern medicine.[79] In 1847, while in a prominent post at the Charité Hospital in Berlin, Virchow co-founded a journal, the *Archiv für pathologische Anatomie und Physiologie und für klinische Medicin*, which served as a forum for the new direction.[80] Building on the work of others, Virchow questioned the speculative, theoretical tendencies of the natural-philosophical school of medicine and its "unchecked propensity to erect hypotheses based on the flimsiest kind of evidence." He posited in its place a method now recognizable as the modern experimental method, one which he and those of a similar mindset now applied in their own research work.[81]

Virchow was not alone in his views, but was part of a progressive scientific movement in the natural sciences. A liberal in politics who had participated in the Berlin street fighting in March 1848, he began publishing a weekly periodical, *Die medicinische Reform* in July 1848 in which he presented his innovative scientific views. The new direction in the natural sciences for men like Virchow did not represent pure science for its own sake, but rather belonged to a part of a liberal program which linked medical enlightenment of the public with democratic political goals. Even after the failure of the 1848 revolution and his dismissal from Berlin for political reasons, Virchow stuck to his agenda, becoming a liberal

---

[79] Lazare Benaroyo, "Rudolf Virchow and the Scientific Approach to Medicine,." *Endeavour* 22, no. 3 (1998): 114.

[80] Andreas W. Daum, *Wissenschaftspopularisierung im 19. Jahrhundert: Bürgerliche Kultur, naturwissenschaftliche Bildung und die deutsche Öffentlichkeit, 1848-1914* (Munich: Oldenbourg, 1998), 446. Publication of the author's 1995 dissertation at the Institut für Neuere Geschichte der Ludwig-Maximilians-Universität, Munich.

[81] Benaroyo, 114. Virchow and scientists like him did not entirely abandon the notion of a unity of nature, at once ridiculing Schelling's natural philosophy and in ways echoing its mystery of the unknowable. A thorough discussion of this question is well beyond the scope of this study; for more see for example Heinrich Schipperges, *Utopien der Medizin. Geschichte und Kritik der ärztlichen Ideologie des 19. Jahrhunderts* (Salzburg, Otto Müller Verlag, 1968) and on the meaning and limitation of Virchow's scientific method, Wolfgang Jacob, "Virchows Begriff der 'naturwissenschaftlichen Methode'–Deutung und Grenzen" in *Wege der Naturforschung 1822-1970 im Spiegel der Versammlungen Deutscher Naturforscher und Ärzte*, Hans Querner and Heinrich Schipperges, eds. (Berlin, Heidelberg: Springer Verlag, 1972).

Prussian parliamentarian after 1858 and a leading member of the Reichstag after 1870.[82]

The frustration of the reform hopes of many liberal scientists in 1848 and the subsequent political reaction led them to concentrate on their scientific efforts, resulting in a strong advance in the natural sciences.[83] Virchow himself, banished from Berlin, accepted a position in Würzburg in 1849, where he continued to advocate the new approach to medicine in the pages of the *Archiv*. The product was his concept of cellular pathology, published in 1858, and which elevated him to the leading figure in the medicine of his time.[84] A major shift in the direction of medicine away from philosophical speculation and empirical observation and toward laboratory-based experimental medicine had begun, a movement that would bring about the development of the modern science of medicine and prove troublesome indeed for the spa physician.

The proceedings of the national congresses of the *Gesellschaft Deutscher Naturforscher und Ärzte* [Society of German Natural Scientists and Physicians] illustrate this development clearly. Founded in 1822, by midcentury the GDNA had grown into an important national forum for the communication of scientific ideas. In the first decades of the society's existence, the congresses showed a noticeable natural-philosophical tendency, but by the middle of the century, a greater experimental-scientific focus became evident.[85] The twenty-ninth assembly of the society, held in Wiesbaden in 1852, included addresses attacking philosophical medicine, reflecting a general trend discernible after 1850, in which gradually, the experimental, physiological approach to medicine achieved dominance.[86]

Thus, in addition to the threat posed by spa physicians' own exaggerated claims of miraculous cures, and from a layman's popular method of water therapy, spa medicine faced a threat from within the medical community as well. The assault on medicine based on natural philosophy, which had begun in the years preceding the 1848 revolutions, and intensified thereafter, posed a considerable threat to spa physicians. Many were aware of the fact that their brand of medicine was behind the

---

82 Daum, *Wissenschaftspopularisierung*, 446 ff.
83 Daum, *Wissenschaftspopularisierung*, 450.
84 Eckart, *Geschichte der Medizin*, p. 274.
85 Heinrich Schipperges, "Repräsentative Eröffnungsreden auf den Naturforscherversammlungen im 19. Jahrhundert" in *Wege der Naturforschung*, 12.
86 Dietrich von Engelhardt, "Naturphilosophie und Wissenschaftstheorie," in *Wege der Naturforschung*, 70.

times, and recognized the need for renewal in order to prevent a loss of credibility and livelihood.

Practitioners in Baden-Baden, perhaps more affected than others by the erosion of their medical reputation by the success of the entertainment branch of the spa enterprise, recognized their peril soonest. In 1854 reports to the Spa Commission on the state of affairs, practicing physicians offered suggestions for how to ensure the continued success of the medical enterprise.[87] Most of their ideas were unimaginative repetitions of the traditional solutions to problems, some of them decades old by now, concerning improvements to the infrastructure and staff, ensuring clean, well-maintained bathtubs, and upgrading the training of staff so that they could better prepare baths according to doctors' orders. In 1854, however, *Badearzt* Saur proved more insightful than his tradition-bound colleagues.[88] In his view, in addition to the usual improvements, it was "of great use" to keep apace of the "advances of science." All practitioners, supported by the spa administration, should "not only utilize what is there [*das Gegebene nutzen*]" but do so "scientifically."[89] As the lengthy report proceeded, it was clear that the author saw the need to cut loose from the past to embrace the new trend in medicine advocated by figures such as Virchow.

Saur's was not a lone voice; many young, dynamic practitioners shared his views. Significantly, these reform-minded doctors jettisoned the term *Badearzt*, preferring to call themselves balneologists, making clear that they practiced balneology or hydrology. The difference was more than semantic. Many senior practitioners clung to the older, philosophical school of medicine. The "young Turks" of the field, however, advocated that their discipline had to advance scientifically if it were to survive at all. In their view, salvation for the field of balneology lay not in a tenacious

---

[87] GLAKa 195/995, reports dated March 18, 1854 (6639) and April 3, 1854 (8092).

[88] Biographical information regarding these practitioners is at best scarce and difficult to locate. Certain patterns are suggested, albeit obliquely, by the handwriting in these reports, which is markedly different among various authors. The authors offering advice of a conventional nature, that is suggesting improvements to facilities and staff, write with handwriting and in a style reminiscent of earlier in the century. Dr. Saur, however, writes using more modern spelling (e.g. *sein* instead of *seyn*) and handwriting of a clearly different and more modern style, implying that he was in fact younger than his colleagues. The evidence is hardly conclusive, but suggests that younger practitioners may have been more progressive than their older counterparts. This will be seen more clearly in the foundation of the *Balneologische Gesellschaft* in 1855 (see below).

[89] GLAKa 195/995, "Mittheilung des zust. Arztes Saur in Baden, über die hiesigen Badeanstalten," April 3, 1854.

loyalty to Romantic natural philosophy, nor in adopting Priessnitz' methods, but in a whole-hearted embrace of progressive trends in academic medicine.

This was a critical moment in the development of the field. Tradition-minded spa physicians remained firmly rooted in medicine inspired by natural philosophy, as discussed in Chapter Three. By the 1850s, however, this school of thought was nearly entirely discredited. Moving ahead from this older view, then, was a matter of life-and-death for the field. If it failed to adapt to the times and adopt current trends in science, hydrotherapy was likely to fall into oblivion. Recognizing this fact, realistic and progressive spa practitioners decided to take action.

On May 1 and 2, 1855, balneologists from across German lands gathered in Berlin for the founding of the *Deutsche Gesellschaft für Hydrologie* [German Society for Hydrology]. The purpose of the *Gesellschaft*, for which the *Balneologische Zeitung* was the mouthpiece, expressly stated in its regulating statutes was "the promotion of hydrology, in the broadest sense of the word, as a science."[90] It admitted only academically-trained physicians as members. The proceedings from this first assembly of the society are a rich source for examining the state of spa medicine at midcentury.

The situation was bleak, and the inaugural address of the society identified many problems. Promotional literature, written mostly for the lay public, did more harm than good, promoting individual spas "almost as industrialists" or "traveling salesmen," evincing almost no interest in science. Physicians outside the field perceived the self-promoting spa doctors as having "a purely pecuniary interest" in their own institutions.[91] The solution to this situation was simple, increased cooperation and dedication to science. An invited paper by a physician from Aachen concurred, contending that the dangers to the discipline were serious. Solutions could be found, however, by turning to proper science based on chemistry and physiology, especially in the published literature; further, cooperation between spas and the application of pressure on governments to establish professorships in balneology would help overcome the problems facing spa medicine. The Aachen practitioner seemed to have in mind, at least in embryo, the formation of a lobbying agency, one that

---

[90] *Die Verhandlungen der deutschen Gesellschaft für Hydrologie während ihrer ersten Generalversammlung zu Berlin am 1. und 2. Mai 1855*, Hofrath Dr. [L.] Spengler, ed. (Wetzlar: Verlag von G. Rathgeber, 1855), 9.

[91] F.J. Behrend, Inaugural Address of the Deutsche Gesellschaft für Hydrologie, in *Die Verhandlungen der deutschen Gesellschaft für Hydrologie während ihrer ersten Generalversammlung zu Berlin am 1. und 2. Mai 1855*, 1-7.

could use professional solidarity to remind the authorities of how financially significant the spas were for state revenues. [92]

The driving force behind the foundation of the *Gesellschaft* was Court Counselor Dr. Ludwig Spengler, a balneologist practicing in Ems. Spengler was a somewhat controversial figure, notoriously combative while paradoxically advocating greater collegiality among balneologists. He envisioned a hydrology based on sound science and saw the need to reform the field that "began empirically"[93] and thereby to "introduce balneology into the ranks of the exact sciences."[94] The mission of the *Gesellschaft,* in short, was to deliver the field from its reputation as a pseudoscience, even as charlatan quackery. While it did not entirely succeed, it did herald a change in the way many practitioners of spa medicine approached research and publication that bore fruit later in the century.[95]

Medical publications in balneology after 1860 exhibited a strong shift in emphasis away from the empirical-philosophical observations, embracing the experimental-scientific approach. That is, it moved with the times. In place of the all-encompassing compendia, the new experimental studies narrowed their focus to such phenomena as the specific content and effect of lithium in Baden-Baden spring water.[96] The new scientific spirit began to make itself felt in the guidebook genre as well. The author of one such general guide for physicians and laypersons tried to make clear how his guide, published in 1862, was different from earlier works. His purpose was to clarify "all obscurities, doubts, mistakes and misuses … as far as the current state of research makes this possible."[97] Further, he endeavored to help raise up balneology "from the shadows of its mysticism and

---

[92] "Was die Balneologie Noth thut. Der Versammlung deutscher Balneologen in Berlin am 1. Mai 1855 eingesendet durch Dr. Diemer in Aachen." *Die Verhandlungen der deutschen Gesellschaft für Hydrologie während ihrer ersten Generalversammlung zu Berlin am 1. und 2. Mai 1855*, 14-17.

[93] Ludwig Spenger, "Was wir bringen" in *Balneologische Zeitung* 1, no. 1 (January 1, 1855): 2.

[94] Spengler, "Was wir bringen," 3.

[95] Hermann Sommer, *Zur Kur nach Ems*, 610.

[96] See, for example, A. Ruef, *Das Lithium und die lithiumhaltigen Quellen von Baden-Baden als wirksames Heilmittel gegen Gicht* (Baden-Baden: Hofbuchhandlung von J.R. Marx, 1862), or D.E.A. Genth, *Untersuchungen über den Einfluß des Wassertrinkens auf den Stoffwechsel* (Wiesbaden, 1856).

[97] Otto Ewich, *Rationelle Balneologie. Praktisches Handbuch über die vorzüglichsten Heilquellen und Curorte für Aerzte und Badereisende* (Berlin: Verlag von August Hirschwald, 1862), i.

superstition" by means of a rational, statistical approach.[98] Clearly, the reform-minded balneologists were intent on becoming part of the new, more scientific medicine. They strove to join the larger, international world of scientific medicine through societies, congresses, and publication, and met with some success.[99]

Still, as detractors of the field made abundantly clear, much of the new "science" of balneology had severe limitations. It remained in essence the same, based not on hard, verifiable data, but rather on unreliable experiences and subjective observations. Balneologists had only adopted the garb of modern science; they attempted to speak the language, shunning terms such as the *Brunnengeist* in favor of lithium, for example, yet they remained unable to substantiate their claims of efficacy or cast off the always faint odor of charlatanism.

What effect the purportedly new balneology may have had on the attitude of the curing public is somewhat difficult to ascertain, but it appears that no immediate change was afoot. Skepticism was surely not erased, as is evidenced in Bismarck's letters of the 1860s and by *Hans-Jörgels Badereise*. Nonetheless, it is possible to come to a more nuanced view of patient reception to the "new" balneology, once again through the use of alternative sources. An examination of popular works from the 1860s, after several years of balneological activity, may shed further light on attitudes toward spa medicine.

Heinrich Hoffmann, known to posterity as the author of the *Struwelpeter*, also wrote a satire of spas and spa doctors, *Das Badeort Salzloch*, literally, "The Spa Salt-Hole," published in 1860.[100] Hoffmann, himself a physician, was little impressed by the new balneology. In a segment devoted to "charlatanism and the art of medicine, "he wrote how "one will never hear from one of the faithful even the most quiet expression of doubt regarding the unconditional reliability and infallibility of the praise" [for the spas] which was "not at all new, and was always so."[101] In the same vein, Hoffmann continued that "a spa curative without a *Badearzt* is the same as

---

98 Ewich, *Rationelle Balneologie*, vii.

99 David Blackbourn, "Taking the Waters': Meeting Places of the Fashionable World." in *The Mechanics of Internationalism. Culture, Society and Politics from the 1840s to the First World War.* Martin H. Geyer and Johannes Paulmann, eds. (Oxford, New York: Oxford University Press, 2001), 440.

100 Heinrich Hoffmann, *Das Badeort Salzloch* (1860). Project Gutenberg Edition, available at http://gutenberg.spiegel.de/hoffmanh/salzloch/Druckversion_salzloch.htm, accessed on June 19, 2003.

101 Hoffmann, Project Gutenberg Edition, Section I, "Einleitung," page 1. http://gutenberg.spiegel.de/hoffmanh/salzloch/Druckversion_salzloch.htm

a marriage without a blessing, namely, a wild one, like a picture without colors, a day without sunshine, like a lost way without plan or path, without a destination or hope for return home, a beastly health-odyssey."[102] These, in turn, were characterized by the character Dr. Goldfischer, whose name declares his motives, even without translation. Even the scientific analyses of the spring waters did not escape the author's wit, as careful reading of the mock-analysis of Salzloch's waters shows that it contained, in a minuscule but no doubt effective quantity, pure clay, pebbles, baregine (an indeterminate substance found in the waters of the French spa Barèges) and human salts, suggestive, of course, of urine.

Clearly skeptical of balneologists' claims to scientific credibility, Hoffmann lampooned their studies. He offered a parody, in which the fictitious Salzloch *Badearzt*, Dr. Polykarpus Gastfenger ("guest catcher"), conducted a study of the spring water "from the perspective of cellular pathology." In the study, Gastfenger placed cancer cells under the microscope immersed in the miraculous waters to study the effects of table salt upon them. After half an hour, the "cancer cells had disappeared, or at least they could not be found," leading to the immediate wide-ranging conclusion that "our spa has a specific dissolving, dispersing and healing force."[103] The effects of the spa waters were supposedly so powerful that, Dr. Gastfenger claimed, "our fleas and bugs are no common fleas and bugs, but are, because of the thermal gases and saline life-transformation, altered and strengthened beings."[104]

Hoffmann, of course, wrote a satire, which cannot be regarded as representative of the views of all physicians, nor should it even be regarded as wholly serious criticism. Nevertheless, that balneology was so remorselessly ridiculed by a physician outside the field does suggest that the efforts to establish the discipline as a science, initially at least, fell far short of what the editors of the *Balneologische Zeitung* could have hoped. The field itself may not have enjoyed a high reputation. At the same time, however, many individual practitioners were well respected as individuals, and were able to make careers in the academic establishment. F.W. Beneke, a balneologist in Nauheim, lectured in balneology at the University of Marburg after 1857; others taught in Vienna, Halle, and a number of

[102] Hoffmann, Project Gutenberg Edition, Section I, "Einleitung," page 3. http://gutenberg.spiegel.de/hoffmanh/salzloch/Druckversion_salzloch.htm
[103] Hoffmann, Project Gutenberg Edition, Part V, "Allgemeine Wirkungen," p. 3. http://gutenberg.spiegel.de/hoffmanh/salzloch/Druckversion_salzloch.htm
[104] Hoffmann, Project Gutenberg Edition, Part V, "Allgemeine Wirkungen," p. 11. http://gutenberg.spiegel.de/hoffmanh/salzloch/Druckversion_salzloch.htm

other universities. Such academic postings were in fact rare, but they illustrate how spa medicine, although marginal, was still within the realm of what was regarded as acceptable academic medicine.[105]

To be fair, one must recall that medicine generally was only beginning to understand the processes of disease in this era, when cholera and tuberculosis were still epidemic. The pioneering work of Louis Pasteur and Robert Koch in the germ theory of disease occurred in the 1870s and the period of modern medicine, associated with bacteriological theory, is generally regarded to have begun in the 1880s.[106] Despite Virchow's advances in physiology, the development of asepsis and anesthesia in surgery, medicine in the 1860s remained decidedly limited in its ability to treat disease. In terms of therapeutic results, hydrotherapy was still little worse (or better) than what other medical techniques had to offer.

An examination of various sources reveal an image of the spa at midcentury, both in its prime, as ever-increasing visitor statistics show, and under attack from several directions. The success of the grand spas in appealing to a wide audience and in creating a cosmopolitan atmosphere of luxury exposed them to charges of harboring vice, hardly suitable for the promotion of health. Baden-Baden, at its zenith of prestige, had to bear the epithet of a "gaming hell," dominated and blemished by vice.

At the same time, many physicians practicing spa medicine grew complacent in their success, and the field stagnated within the confines of Romantic medicine. This backwardness combined with promotional literature that promised impossibly effective cures to undermine the spas' aspiration to be places of serious curing. In this atmosphere, the innovations of a layman, Vincenz Priessnitz, entered to challenge spa physicians' assertions of authority. Priessnitz' own success, and that of his imitators, cast further into doubt the already tenuous position that formal medical expertise was necessary in order to tap the salutary properties of water. The association of water-therapy with a layman only served to reinforce a perception that all "water-doctors" were alike: amateurs, not scientists.

Spa medicine, then, for all its apparent success, was in a time of transitional crisis. Certainly patients came to the spas, and indeed took the waters for healing. Crowded waiting rooms in physicians practices

---

[105] H. v. Mettenheim, "Vom Denken und Handeln der Badeärzte in den Jahren 1850-1898 nach Briefen," *Zeitschrift für angewandte Bäder- und Klimaheilkunde*, 25 (1978): 318-325. See also Joachim Moerchel, *Die Nassauischen Badeärzte.*

[106] L. Margaret Barnett, review of *Making Medicine Scientific: John Burdon Sanderson and the Culture of Victorian Science* by Terrie M. Romano, *Journal of the American Medical Association* 289 (June 25,2003): 3312.

indicate that many did in fact seek medical counsel for their ailments. But spa physicians, now bearing the new self-conferred title of balneologists, still did not command the authority they had always sought: to be regarded and respected, beyond all doubt, as experts. Patients continued either to attempt to cure themselves with the waters, or perhaps more aggravating to a resident balneologist, followed advice from their own personal physician back home, spurning the expert who specialized in the use of the springs. Still, they remained ambivalent about their doctors. Criticism was far less caustic than earlier in the century, and yet, doctors were far from being regarded as nearly omnipotent authorities in the battle against disease. As the spa world suggests, middle-class patients consulted physicians, but also well knew that there was not much they could do.

The response to this situation lay not in embracing the alternative offered by Priessnitz and his followers, but precisely in the opposite direction. If spa physicians were to survive and be perceived as more than "water doctors," they needed a new name and a new image; they became balneologists, and thereby proclaimed their embrace of cutting-edge approaches to medicine. Their rejection of alternative medicine was absolute and uncompromising. Instead, they sought to secure and solidify their position within the medical establishment, and longed to be respected by their colleagues in the academy and by patients alike.

At the critical juncture of the mid-nineteenth century, when the development of modern medical science began to take shape, balneologists were clear in their minds that they were and wished to remain part of the academy. In subsequent decades, from the 1870s onward, medicine underwent yet greater transformations. Prevention and therapy, at last, grew more effective with greater understanding of disease processes. With the deepening of medical understanding, greater specialization into specialties and subspecialties became the new trend in medical education and practice. Building on the foundations set in the 1850s, balneologists redefined themselves to meet this new development, now seeking to be recognized as specialists and laying claim authority and prestige on this basis. How successful they were in this endeavor is discussed in the next chapter.

CHAPTER FIVE

STRUGGLE FOR SURVIVAL: CURING VICE AND ENLISTING SCIENCE

On September 15, 1871, the Russian novelist and long-time resident Ivan Turgenev, wrote in a letter from Baden-Baden: "Everything bears the mark of the end, of dissolution."[1] The year for Baden-Baden, if not the end of an era, marked the beginning of an uncertain future. The Franco-Prussian War had driven away French visitors, so important to the prosperity of the previous decades. Worse, however, in the following year, 1872, the ultimate *rien ne vas plus* sounded, the result of sustained opposition to gambling that at last succeeded in closing the casino. The handwriting had long been on the wall, and the end of the reign of the roulette wheel was only a question of time after 1867, when the North German Confederation passed a ban on the risky pastime throughout its territory, effective as of 1870, at a time when the prospect of the inclusion of Baden in a unified German state under Prussian leadership lay near. The disappearance of the casino, both as a social focal point of the grand spas, as Turgenev and many others felt, and as a steadfast cash cow threatened to destroy everything the spas had come to represent. Elegance, cosmopolitan sophistication, and refined amusement, it was feared, would vanish with the roulette wheel. More concretely, aficionados feared that denied these intangible assets, Baden-Baden and other spas would be condemned to decline and ruin. To some, the progression seemed simple: no casino, no money, no guests.

[1] Ivan Turgenev, letter from September 15, 1871, cited in Rolf Gustav Haebler, *Geschichte der Stadt Baden und des Kurortes Baden-Baden*, Second Edition, (Baden-Baden: Verlag Dr. Willy Schmidt, 1969) 2: 131. Turgenev lived in Baden-Baden from 1864-1871, moving then to Paris. As one popular legend of the town would have it, he told Dostoevsky in an 1867 argument over literature and the latter's unpaid debt of fifty *thaler*, "I have permanently settled here in Baden-Baden, and no longer regard myself as a Russian, but as a German, and that I am proud of it!" See Haebler, *Geschichte der Stadt Baden und des Kurortes* 2: 100.

Others, seeing things from a different vantage point than Turgenev, the permanent *Kurgast* for leisure, could smell opportunity. Removing the key source of vice they saw as a chance to revitalize and rededicate the spa and to recover its core purpose of curing. This prospect made many, including all balneologists, jubilant. The healing waters themselves, and the specialists in their use, would be the centerpiece of the spas, while charges of frivolity and decadence would finally be silenced. The chance had arrived for the fulfillment of the dream the German Society for Hydrology had set out in 1855: by moving bravely forward, balneology would be regarded not as antiquated Romantic mysticism, but as serious medicine, the crisis of credibility solved. Without the casino, not only could the spa, and balneology, survive, but indeed they would blossom with renewed vigor.

This was not all a pipedream, but rather a realistic assessment of the state of affairs. Austrian spas had never hosted the kind of wild gaming seen in German lands, and France had banned games of chance in 1837. In each, spas had survived and even thrived.[2] Karlsbad and Marienbad in Austria, Vichy and Plombières in France were compelling examples of how a spa could do well without a wagering public. Still, the transformation that exhilarated physicians filled administrators and entrepreneurs with anxiety as they imagined their ledgers without gamblers' gulden.

They could not claim that the end of gaming had taken them by surprise, however. As early as 1847, the *Morgenblatt*, discussed at length speculations that the demise of the casino might be near, and that Baden-Baden and other casinos might have to find other means of support.[3] Discussions such as these and even vociferous critiques of games of chance that appeared even earlier in the pages of the *Morgenblatt* and other periodicals, such as Emma Niendorf's from 1845 (see Chapter Four), were far from the only sign that the casino was under siege. In January 1843, the Badenese diet debated a motion to prohibit the casino as a

---

[2] It is true, however, that after 1837, the French gambling public then traveled to spas abroad, most frequently to Baden-Baden. A notable exception to the gambling prohibition in France was Aix-les-Bains. When the town that had belonged to Savoy was annexed in 1860, the French government allowed the casino to continue. See Douglas Peter Mackaman, *Leisure Settings: Bourgeois Culture, Medicine and the Spa in Modern France* (Chicago and London: University of Chicago Press, 1998), 48, 58.

[3] "Badener Zustände," *Morgenblatt für gebildete Leser*, No. 152 (June 26, 1847): 605 ff.

manifestation of "sin and shame."[4] The motion failed, but this was far from the last time parliamentary bodies deliberated on the question. The Diet of the Germanic Confederation considered banning casinos in 1845, but decided to allow their continued existence. The Revolution of 1848, however, brought a much more tangible threat. In January 1849, the Frankfurt National Assembly passed legislation that was to prohibit casinos throughout the German Reich as of May 1 of that year.[5] The casino in Baden-Baden was in fact closed for a time, but with the failure of the Revolution and the arrival of Prussian troops in the Grand Duchy in July 1849, the Frankfurt legislation became inoperative.

The restoration of the old regime and the old gaming order did not quell the strong opposition to the pernicious pastime. In 1861, the Badenese Grand Duke Friedrich declared the casino concession would not be renewed when it expired in 1867, a date later postponed to 1870.[6] The North German Confederation's ban for 1870 applied to Wiesbaden and Ems since the principality of Nassau, in which these spas were located, entered the Confederation in 1866 along with Frankfurt, Schleswig-Holstein and other territories. As long as Baden remained independent, the spa could still hope to fight with the Grand Ducal government for another lease on life for its casino. The unification of Germany in 1871, however, dashed any such hopes, as the ban valid in the Northern German Confederation was to apply to the entire German Reich. One final extension was granted to allow the spa town to set its affairs in order, but the date for the final closure of the casino was set for October 31, 1872.

The loss of their casinos meant above all a financial crisis for Baden-Baden and Wiesbaden, which collected much of their operating funds directly from the gambling franchise. Smaller spas, even those without their own lucrative casinos were threatened as well, since gambling profits flowed through state agencies into subsidies for smaller, less frequented spas. The Badenese government, for example, redistributed some of the proceeds from Baden-Baden to the salines in nearby Rappenau for infrastructure development and maintenance.[7] Prohibition meant belt-tightening and readjustment for the spa industry as a whole.

State authorities, aware of the crisis the decision would unleash, initiated appropriate measures to ease the transition from dependence on casino revenue. The plan for Baden-Baden involved a deep reorganization

---

[4] Motion put before the Badenese Diet, January 3, 1843, by Freiherr von Andlaw, cited in Haebler, *Geschichte der Stadt Baden und des Kurortes*, 2: 81.
[5] Haebler, *Geschichte der Stadt Baden und des Kurortes*, 2: 84.
[6] Haebler, *Geschichte der Stadt Baden und des Kurortes*, 2: 125.
[7] Haebler, *Geschichte der Stadt Baden und des Kurortes*, 2: 126.

of both the financial and administrative structure of the spa. In a significant departure from the past, after 1871 the town authorities were integrated into the management of the spa. No longer was Baden-Baden administered directly from Karlsruhe. The Spa Commission, established in 1805 as a department of the Ministry of the Interior, was dissolved and replaced with a local Cure Committee, composed of representatives of the city council, and chaired by the mayor of the town. The Badenese Ministry of the Interior retained a general supervisory role, but day-to-day management of the spa, as well as the responsibility for the success or failure, including its fiscal management, fell to this new Cure Committee. The town, in this moment of looming crisis, at last received the authority it had coveted for decades.

Authority came at a price, however, and finances, too, underwent a corresponding fundamental shift. Until 1871, operating funds for the spa, mostly derived from casino gambling, were administered from Karlsruhe. After 1871, the Grand Ducal government provided a substantial subsidy from a trust fund in which it had put aside the revenues from the final years of gaming. So, for example in 1877 the spa received 77,150 marks in subsidies from the capital. Yet this was far from the complete operating budget -- the city of Baden-Baden was required to produce 120,000 M in subsidies the same year. This was over half of the total revenue for the year, with the remainder of the 222,000 M budget coming from other sources such as fees for amusements and the *Kurtaxe.* [8] This paltry level of support meant that the spa would have to sink or swim on its own.

The casino might be closed, but could gambling, so intrinsic to the spa experience, actually be entirely banned? If, as Dostoevsky and other critics of the “gaming hell” so clearly indicated, one of the main attractions of Baden-Baden was the promise of quick riches, and the rich and powerful were particularly fond of this “noble pastime,” was a ban even possible? Wagering guests not only left their money behind on the green tables of the Conversation House, but spent lavishly in hotels, restaurants, and local businesses. The Cure Committee, representing local commercial interests, was well aware of the risk involved in completely losing this lucrative commerce. Consequently, there was selective enforcement of the ban on gambling, with the greatest exceptions being made for the most affluent and prestigious individuals.

In 1858, a racetrack was built in Iffezheim, just a few miles outside of Baden-Baden proper. Conceived as a profitable enterprise that would bring

---

[8] Stadtarchiv Baden Baden Signatur 20-17-153, (hereafter referred to in short form as StA BB 20-17-153). “Rechenschaftsberichte der Kurverwltungskasse, 1877+.”

greater cosmopolitan sophistication to the spa, it was a success for its investors, who included Edouard Benazet, the holder of the casino franchise. Closure of the casino proved to be a boon for the races at Iffezheim. In the fall of 1872, a group of private individuals, led by Prince Karl Egon von Fürstenberg, founded the International Club, a private organization of racing enthusiasts, who established their clubhouse in an elegant villa on the road to Iffezheim.[9] The club was responsible for organizing the races as well as the maintenance of the track, and received along with this authority considerable subsidies from the city. Members included local business and tradesmen, who paid annual membership dues to support its activities, apparently not always eagerly or even willingly. The club was, however, clearly dominated by the higher orders from outside of town. The board of directors consisted entirely of noblemen, and in 1907 included names such as Graf Lehndorff, Graf August von Bismarck, and Prinz Hans von Hohenlohe.[10]

Their passion does not appear to have been limited to appreciation of the graceful speed of thoroughbreds. One can only speculate what occurred within the confines of the private clubhouse, but it is safe to assume that members continued to indulge privately in games of chance as they once had publicly in the Conversation House. Private high-stakes games of faro between important gentlemen were something to which law enforcement could easily turn a blind eye. Yet evidence suggests that the International Club and the races at Iffezheim were not subject to strict enforcement on the ban on gambling outside the clubhouse, either. Municipal police records on the maintenance of order at the track report in remarkably similar words year after year how bookies were observed working at the races. Curiously, there are no references to any arrests for this offense. On the other hand, a master butcher was arrested and fined for riding his bicycle down the road to the track in 1890, a habit that had been the subject of complaints from important individuals who found fast-riding cyclists to be a menace to those taking a leisurely stroll.[11]

Clearly, some forms of gambling among luminaries in the spa were tolerated at an official level. Yet the spa could not entirely flaunt the prohibition on gambling. The casino in the Conversation House was in fact shut down on October 31, 1872, but low-stakes gambling continued,

---

[9] Johann Loeser, *Geschichte der Stadt Baden* (Baden-Baden: Sommermeyer, 1891), 416.

[10] StA BB 26-15-184. "Subventionierung Baden-Iffezheimer Pferderennen, Stadtrat, Kursachen. 1906-18."

[11] GLAKa 339/1344. "Handhabung der öffentlichen Sicherheit und Ordnung bei den Pferderennen zu Iffezheim. 1858-1873; 1883-1893." Police report from 1890.

although in subdued form. How to handle this situation generated a fair amount of correspondence between spas, with Baden-Baden consulting Bad Ems in 1891, for example, about fees for card games; other letters suggested that games played for prize money, as in Bad Homburg near Frankfurt, be introduced in Baden.[12] The question revolved around the distinction, never clear, between "games of chance," that were prohibited, and "games of skill" with a prize paid to the winner, that were allowed. The same rooms that once housed the roulette wheel and faro tables, after 1872, were set up as billiard and card rooms, where whist and other games were played with official cards, sold at a premium price. Betting on these games did in fact continue, although hardly at the level it once had, and gaming of this kind never produced more than modest sums for the spa. Gambling became a strictly private (and legally dubious) matter. For those who wished to gamble for high stakes, the horse races seem to have replaced the roulette wheel. Those who came to Baden-Baden solely to gamble could still do so, if under somewhat different circumstances. But the casino and all it meant was gone. Turgenev sold his furniture, his house, and left Baden-Baden for good in 1872.

The dynamic center of the spa, the Conversation House with its casino, had been subdued, transformed from something thrilling, if controversial, into a somewhat sedate meeting point. Even if gambling in the spa did continue privately, the spa no longer drew massive revenues from it, and it did not occur in the center of the spa. With the heart of the spa removed, many wondered how it could survive. Addressing these and more general questions, the physician Karl Frech published in 1870 a statistical analysis of the habits of the spa-going public in Baden-Baden from 1858 to 1869.[13] He concluded that Baden-Baden did in fact host more than its share of pleasure-seekers, making it more a *Luxusbad* [Luxury resort] than a *Kurort* [place of curing]. In an environment in which most other spas had already closed their casinos, dependence on the casino, Frech sternly cautioned, would bring calamity. The solution he advocated was one that had been predicted in the pages of the *Morgenblatt* in 1847, that deliverance from crisis and upheaval was at hand in the spas' healing waters:

---

[12] StA BB 20-14-1, "Einrichtung und Betrieb des Spielsaals im Kurhaus, 1872-1914" See for example letters from the administration of Bad Homburg to the Cure Committee, dated September 25, 1874, from the Cure Committee to Bad Ems, dated December 9, 1891, with a response dated December 11, 1891.

[13] Karl Frech, *Der Kurort Baden-Baden, Ein Beitrag zur Geschichte des heutigen Badewesens* (Karlsruhe: Chr. Fr. Müller'sche Hofbuchhandlung, 1870).

> [W]ith or without the casino, the spa can look to a future in which the healing springs, the pleasant surroundings and the natural amenities will again assume the main role that has only temporarily been taken from them [by the casino]. With a clever eye toward this future, the time of the golden rain has been used for preparations. Of all the accomplishments of the famous Doctor Guggert [one of the leading spa physicians in Baden-Baden at the time–KW], surely not the least is that has been promoting the curative facilities with tireless energy.[14]

Other spas, such as Wiesbaden evidently reached the same conclusion. Following the example of smaller, yet successful, spas, the grand spas would seek their fortune, indeed, their survival, in emphasizing medicine and healing.

This shift to curing seemed a logical and natural solution. Frech contended, with the support of hard numbers, that although there was some truth to the reputation that the grand spas were not sought out for their waters, curing had always gone on in the shadow of the casino. The challenge, then, was not to create a new curing environment, but to make curing the focal point of the spa. For spa physicians like Frech, this seemed to be a return to the natural and proper purpose of the spa, and the authorities, responsive to pressure to do something about the vice associated with gambling, were of a similar mind. Although contemporary sources asserted that the shift in emphasis was "the wish of His Royal Majesty, Grand Duke Friedrich,"[15] it was likely because of the influence of physicians that Frech's vision for the future of Baden-Baden prevailed after 1870. The new Baden-Baden was to remain full of grandeur, but most of all it would be a respectable place of leisure and of serious curing.

The partial suppression of gambling brought the spa's central paradox back into prominence. Was the spa primarily a place for relaxation and amusement, or was it about serious curing? This round of discussion produced a firmer resolution to the eternal question. Lip-service was paid once again to the idea of complementarity: curing and amusement were not in conflict. During the middle decades of the nineteenth century however, curing, it was generally conceded, had been overshadowed by amusement. The correct balance was now to be restored. After 1870, the effort was not to reinvent the spa, but to return it to a healthy relationship

---

[14] "Badener Zustände," *Morgenblatt für gebildete Leser* no. 153 (July 28, 1847): 611.

[15] *Das Friedrichbad in Baden-Baden. Beschreibung des Baues und Anleitung zum Gebrauche der Bäder und der Trinkkur, nebst Badeordnung* (Baden-Baden, D.M. Marx'sche Hofbuchhandlung, 1878), 1. See also Loeser, *Geschichte der Stadt Baden*, 351 ff.

between the two parts of its being. Spa physicians were in agreement: medicine and leisure (in moderation) were far from contradictory; they complemented one another and belonged together. With the prohibition on gambling, balneologists could feel that they had recovered the soul of the spa, and it again would emphasize what was most important: the art and science of healing.

This shift in emphasis can be seen concretely in the projects undertaken by the new Cure Committee for the development and promotion of the spa. The first major project was one which many spa physicians had called for since the 1850s: a new steam bath facility offering luxury and medical sophistication. A plan drafted by Frech had been in circulation since 1861, but no action on it was taken.[16] With the disappearance of the casino imminent, however, Frech's plan appeared more attractive as a means to draw new and retain loyal old guests in Baden-Baden. A new design was drafted, the foundation laid in 1869, and the imposing Friedrichsbad, named after the Grand Duke Friedrich I, was opened to the public in 1877.

This new bathhouse was conceived as part of the solution to the impending crisis threatened by the disappearance of the casino. When completed, it possessed features that, it was hoped, would appeal to visitors. First, the Friedrichsbad was to be a state-of-the-art medical facility, offering the newest hydrotherapeutic techniques, including individual bathing cabinets, a range of shower and steam therapies, as well as massage and physiotherapy options. As one contemporary source announced, "with the construction of the Friedrichsbad, a facility that meets all the demands of modern balneotherapy, our city is given back its natural destiny to be and remain a place of healing [*Kurort*]."[17]

The Friedrichsbad was designed to be more than simply a rational medical choice; it appealed also to the senses and to emotions. The city chronicler Loeser wrote with pride, "a thousand years of rubble and junk have been removed … [and] 1600 years later [after the Romans], on the same spot, a monumental structure rises up, a replica of the Roman *thermae*, equipped with the newest and best advances and equipment in balneological therapy."[18] Housed in a strikingly massive edifice that evoked princely grandeur and historical continuity, the keystone of Baden-Baden's new image was designed to impress as a magnificent, modern-day Roman bath. The façade was (and is today) resplendent with sculpted

[16] Karl Frech, *Entwurf für das Neue Dampfbad in Baden-Baden* (Scotzniovsky'sche Buchdruckerei, Baden, 1861).
[17] Loeser, *Geschichte der Stadt Baden*, 351.
[18] Loeser, *Geschichte der Stadt Baden*, 351.

busts of Hadrian and Marcus Aurelius, alongside Grand Duke Friedrich of Baden and the recently deceased Karl Frech next to Hippocrates and Paracelsus. Visitors could imagine that they were bathing much as the Romans had. Even the choice of location was evocative. Beneath the modern bath, the ruins of the Roman *thermae* of Aurelia Aquensis, built in the reign of Marcus Aurelius, were carefully preserved and exhibited in a new museum. The Friedrichsbad, then, brought dreams of the venerable Roman Empire to the modern German one, spinning a myth of continuity borne through the centuries by the same warm waters that had bathed Hadrian. Imperial grandeur was enlisted to promote taking the waters. A visit to the spa was no longer to be seen as a trip into the world of high-rolling dandies, but a sojourn in the glory and power that was Rome, amidst the marvels of nineteenth-century German science and knowledge.

A sense of German imperial pride, then, was coupled with medicine to attract visitors to the spa, hoping they would not miss the casino or what it represented. The link between nationalism and medicine was not as arbitrary or promotionally calculating as it may at first seem. Although concrete progress in curing diseases and illness remained limited in the nineteenth century, the high status of German medicine was a source of immense pride. An increasingly wide public kept abreast developments in the medical and other natural sciences through popular journals; admiration for the achievements of German luminaries such as Robert Koch was genuine.[19] Medical discoveries made by German researchers were a source of patriotic pride, and as a result, advances in the science of medicine bolstered medical authority.[20] Health and hygiene came to be linked not only with personal development and virtue, but indeed with national greatness. To be clean in mind and body, to be a healthy individual, was seen as a duty to the fatherland. Taking good care of one's health was, in effect, part of being a good German as well.[21]

---

[19] For a full discussion of the popularization of science, see Andreas W. Daum, *Wissenschafttspopularisierung in 19. Jahrhundert: Bürgerliche Kultur, naturwissenschaftliche Bildung und die deutsche Öffentlichkeit, 1848-1914* (Munich: Oldenbourg, 1998); Gudrun Wolfschmidt, ed., *Popularisierung der Naturwissenschaften*. (Berlin: Diepholz, 2002).

[20] Paul Weindling, "Bourgeois values, doctors and the state: the professionalization of medicine in Germany, 1848-1933," in David Blackbourn and Richard J. Evans, eds., *The German Bourgeoisie. Essays on the German middle class from the late eighteenth to the early twentieth century* (London and New York: Routledge, 1991), 217-218.

[21] See Alfons Labisch, "Doctors, Workers and the Scientific Cosmology of the Industrial World: The Social Construction of 'Health' and the 'Homo Hygienicus," *Journal of Contemporary History* 20 (1985), 599-615; Manuel Frey, *Der reinliche*

Symbolically important as it may have been, a technically advanced and architecturally impressive bathhouse which touted national pride could not stand alone. Science also needed to be enlisted to support its effectiveness. The spa leadership was aware that Baden-Baden's reputation as a serious place of curing was suspect. "The dubious fortune of a public casino," had established the image of the town as a luxurious playground for the rich [*Luxusbad*], rarely sought out for its waters.[22] The administration was intent on drawing the town out from under the shadow of the casino, and to revive its reputation not only for luxury, but for healing. To this end, a concerted publicity campaign was undertaken to spread the word of the new Baden-Baden.

In the 1870s and 1880s, the Friedrichsbad stood at the center of this publicity effort. Announcements were sponsored in newspapers throughout Germany and abroad to herald the opening. An information pamphlet, reprinted from an 1877 medical journal article, went to press in 1878 for distribution to physicians.[23] It touted the new bathhouse as "an exemplary facility, as in no other spa," describing in specific detail each of the types of baths available, including electrical baths in copper tubs, various forms of shower and immersion baths, plus inhalation rooms, and saunas. An expanded version of this text appeared also in 1878 in a richly bound festschrift which was to make clear to all: Baden-Baden was a place of curing.[24] The article and pamphlet acknowledged the disrepute that the casino had brought upon the town, but then concluded by presenting a glorious new vision of the future:

> Gambling had brought to our spa a false reputation, and had pushed our mineral springs somewhat into the background. The visitor frequency since the closure of the casino, however, amply proves that the reputation of our

---

Bürger, Kritische Studien zur Geschichtswissenschaft vol. 119, Helmut Berding, Jürgen Kocka, Hans-Peter Ullmann, Hans-Ulrich Wehler, eds. (Göttingen: Vanderhoeck & Ruprecht, 1996); Michael Hau, "The Holistic Gaze in German Medicine, 1890-1930," *Bulletin of the History of Medicine* 74 (2000): 495-524; Martina Kessel, "The 'Whole Man:' The Longing for a Masculine World in Nineteenth-Century Germany," *Gender & History* 15, no. 1 (April, 2003): 1-31.

[22] Karl Frech, *Der Kurort Baden-Baden. Ein Beitrag zur Geschichte und Statistik des heutigen Badwesens* (Karlsruhe, Chr. Fr. Müller'sche Buchhandlung, 1870), 3.

[23] StA BB 20-13-3, "Friedrichsbad Brochüren." "Das Friedrichsbad in Baden-Baden," first published in *Ärztliche Mittheilungen aus Baden*, no. 23 and 24 (1877).

[24] *Das Friedrichsbad in Baden-Baden. Beschreibung des Baues und Anleitung zum Gebrauche der Bäder und der Trinkkur, nebst Badeordnung* (Baden-Baden, D.R. Marx'sche Hofbuchhandlung, 1878).

> healing springs has come again into its own. This new exemplary facility will contribute significantly to this end. The long-famous warm saline springs of Baden, a precious jewel of the town and the entire country, must be rejuvenated in this new form and use that lends them a credibility, to which even the greatest doubters will be converted.[25]

Finally, the authors invoked Goethe and implicitly, the memory of a past in which Baden-Baden's waters were paramount:

> Wunderwirkend strömt die Welle
> Strömt der heiße Dampf der Quelle
> Muth wird freier, Blut wird neuer
> Heil dem Wasser, Heil dem Feuer![26]
>
> [Working wonders the wave is streaming
> Streaming the hot steam of the spring
> Feelings become freer, blood newer
> Hail water! Hail fire!]

A second publication of a different nature appeared in 1879 to continue the effort to recast Baden-Baden's image as a *Kurort* distinguished for its springs. The newly appointed Grand Ducal *Badearzt,* Franz Heiligenthal, edited a history of the city and the springs of Baden-Baden, a well-written historical narrative based in archival research. The history, however, was written to convey a message, a clear echo of Frech's program, and concluded with the assessment that Baden-Baden would certainly have a bright future as a place of serious curing. The *Luxusbad* past, in which the casino was dominant and curing was relegated to the background, was portrayed as an aberration. Liberated from the burden of gaming, the author asserted, the spa would return to its natural state as a place of healing at the forefront of modern, technical, and scientific medicine.[27]

A medical guidebook published in 1886 advanced the redefinition of the spa still further. This volume, compiled by a committee of doctors on behalf of the Baden Association of Physicians, no longer addressed the apparently solved problem of the casino, but focused entirely on the practice of medicine in the spa. Intended to assist general practitioners throughout Germany in deciding which patients to send to Baden-Baden, it offered "colleagues the scientific basis for the various therapeutic media

---

[25] Sta BB 20-13-3, "Das Friedrichsbad in Baden-Baden."

[26] Goethe, *Faust,* excerpted in "Das Friedrichsbad in Baden-Baden."

[27] Franz Heiligenthal, ed., *Geschichte der Stadt Baden und ihrer Bäder, nach amtlichen Quellen* (Karlsruhe: G. Braun'sche Hofbuchdruckerei, 1879).

and techniques" to be found there.[28] The authors were attempting to break new ground, presenting the latest scientific knowledge to replace outdated guides, and to fill the gap left by popular guides that simply enumerated the therapies but failed to explain them in a manner satisfactory to those considering prescribing a cure. The guidebook presented balneology as one of the growing specializations in medicine. In order to be at all accessible, not only to educated and interested laymen, but indeed to non-specialist physicians, balneology required expert elucidation.

To spread the word of the new Baden-Baden, promotional efforts targeted at physicians alone would have been inadequate, as the Cure Committee was evidently aware. A substantial number of guests selected a spa on their own, basing their decision on a given locale's reputation, and so for the general public, a slightly different approach was in order. Administrative records show that beginning no later than 1873, and likely earlier, the Cure Committee sponsored the publication of articles flattering to Baden-Baden and managed to place them in numerous local and national newspapers across Germany and abroad.[29] The authors were paid an honorarium directly from the administration for each article they published regarding the spa. In many cases, they were written by the editor-in-chief of the *Badeblatt*, in other cases by journalists working on commission. The members of the Cure Committee did not write these articles directly, nonetheless, they must be regarded as press releases. They reliably and consistently repeated the same themes. The weather did in fact change from time to time, and sometimes the concerts and theatre performances were better than others. Be this as it may, Baden-Baden was *always* a pleasant, safe, and enjoyable place to visit, growing steadily in popularity and renown for its atmosphere, its physicians, and its waters. Respectable people of all kinds were to be seen there, although the press releases never missed the opportunity to trumpet the visits of especially prominent personalities, such as members of the Imperial or other royal households. The advertising function of the *Kurlisten*, celebrating the

[28] Dr. [no first name given] v. Corval, "Einleitung," in Baumgartner, Corval, Frey, Hoffmann, Schliep and Schneider, *Baden-Baden und seine Kurmittel* (Baden-Baden, C. Wild Hofbuchhandlung, 1886), i.

[29] StA BB 20-13-1. "Auswärtige Presse, Remunerations-Bewilligungen von Herrn Damance," StA BB 20-13-9, "Auswärtige Presse, Von Herrn Redakteur Harder geschriebenen Artikel, zur Versendung in auswärtigen Zeitungen," and StA BB 20-13-14, "Auswärtige Presse: Korrespondenzen des Herrn St. in auswärtige Zeitungen, 1900+." Detailed records of articles sponsored by the Cure Committee survive in the archives for the period after 1873, but suggest that this advertising strategy was employed previously, if less intensively.

arrival of eminent visitors, was transferred to a national audience through the press. Readers throughout Germany and abroad could now read about the new Baden-Baden and its reputable environs in their crowded hometowns and imagine, so the sponsors hoped, a salutary sojourn in the spa surrounded by beauty and respectability.

Regular press releases were supplemented by full-page advertisements and flyers that stressed both the tangible and intangible assets of the spa. In this regard, Wiesbaden, perhaps motivated by a desire to surpass Baden-Baden in popularity, took the initiative, publishing in 1877 a large format supplement in the *Norddeutsche Allgemeine Zeitung*. The supplement was clear in its agenda to highlight the advanced medical therapies offered in the spa, followed only in the last part of the advertisement by opportunities for amusement and recreation. Wiesbaden, having lost its own casino, was evidently following a similar promotional agenda.

The Wiesbaden insert was found, apparently with alarm, by Dr. Fritz Heiligenthal, who sent it with dispatch to the Cure Committee. The committee quickly responded, noting that the advertisement had appeared in "all the larger German newspapers," and requesting that Heiligenthal provide pertinent information for drafting a similar prospectus for Baden-Baden as soon as possible.[30] The product appeared within a matter of weeks. The large-format insert followed a similar pattern, emphasizing Baden-Baden's scientifically-based therapeutic options, including what would soon be available in the new Friedrichsbad. Thereafter, similar large-format advertisements, as well as smaller, less expensive advertisements, regularly appeared in national newspapers and popular magazines, for example in the *Frankfurter Zeitung* and the mass-circulation magazine, *Die Gartenlaube*, always emphasizing the power of the healing waters, the technical sophistication of the spa's facilities, and of course, how pleasant a sojourn in Baden-Baden could be.

Illustrated brochures and posters singing the praises of the spa were an additional publicity tool. The content of these flyers remained consistent from the 1870s to 1914. Printed in large formats, on high-quality paper, these color prints often included artwork that either highlighted the natural beauty of the region, the bathing facilities, or both. The accompanying text emphasized the curative value of a visit to Baden-Baden. For example, an 1897 full-color flier praises the Friedrichsbad as "unique in its completeness and elegance," continuing to list seventeen different medical

---

[30] StA BB 20-17-155, "Curörtliche Verhältnisse, 1877-1888." Letter from the Cure Committee to Dr. Franz Heiligenthal, May 17, 1877.

options available in the spa, ranging from "all forms of showers and baths" and "cold-water and fango therapy" in the Friedrichsbad, to a clinic for the treatment of morphine addiction.[31] By the early 1900s, brochures added the latest advance in hydrotherapy, the exploitation of mineral waters containing radioisotopes, while not neglecting to mention in the same sentence that the "world-famous waters" had been in use "already in the days of the Romans."[32] Significantly, the English-language version of this brochure, issued at the same time for tourist offices abroad, placed greater emphasis on tourist attractions such as the castle and the Black Forest. Advertising of the medical facilities, it seems, was targeted toward the German audience.

These general interest brochures and posters were distributed by the thousands in the spa, of course, but also in train stations, the lounges of steamships, even in other resorts on the French Riviera in wintertime. Clearly, the purpose was to attract the traveling public to Baden-Baden, and evidently, emphasizing cutting-edge curing was regarded as an important means to this end for the German public. This can also be observed in guidebooks for the general public, which did not fail to emphasize medicine in the spa. As the editors of the 1886 guide pointed out, however, these generally did little more than list the therapies available, without providing detail as to techniques for the application of the waters.[33] In this respect, these guides are reminiscent of present-day advertisements for prescription drugs, urging a nineteenth-century reader in effect to "ask your doctor about fango therapy." The marvels of late nineteenth-century balneology were proclaimed and showcased, the praises of the specialists sung, but specifics were omitted and left in the domain of experts.

This disappearance of medical "insider information" from popular guidebooks was a general trend. As discussed in the previous two chapters, guidebooks until the 1850s and even the 1860s often provided the general public with step-by-step instructions on how to use the waters effectively, explanations of the medical understanding of why they

---

[31] StA BB 20-13-8, "Herstellung von Herstellung von Führern, Reklameplakate, Prospekte, Umgebungskarten, Klischees, etc. 1893+," Illustrated brochure "Baden-Baden," dated August 24, 1897.

[32] StA BB 20-13-8, Illustrated Brochure issued by the City Information Office, Baden-Baden, undated, ca. 1913.

[33] See for example *Taschenbuch für Badereisende. Jahrbuch der Bäder, Curorte, Heilanstalten 1873*, 5. verbesserte Auflage (Berlin: Denicke's Verlag, 1873); Elise Püttner, *Nordostdeutsche Städte und Landschaften, No. 1: Ostseebad Zoppot bei Danzig* (Danzig: A.W. Kafemann, 1887).

worked, all together with stern warnings not to attempt any of this curing without the strict supervision of a qualified physician. By the 1880s, such information is conspicuously absent. One guide, *Wie Soll der Patient im Kurort Leben*, published in 1909 did continue the stern warning, that "the ill person, as always, should live in spas following the directions of his physician precisely,"[34] but this was an isolated case. The authors of other guides, evidently, did not believe such a warning was necessary, trusting, perhaps, that patients would indeed ask their physician.

This disappearance of warnings is indicative of a larger trend. Medicine by this period had grown much more complicated, and much more the domain of specialists as specialization replaced the earlier ideal of general *Bildung*.[35] The popularization of science may have spread the word of the wonders of German discoveries, yet the real secrets lay in the hands of the experts in academic medicine. Few educated readers needed to be reminded not to attempt to practice medicine on themselves, much as today a magazine such as *Popular Mechanics* may tout the marvels of the latest microprocessor-controlled engine, but few would attempt to repair one themselves.

More specific literature was now available to physicians who might prescribe a spa cure to patients. One example, released in 1909 to "physicians and persons who request scientific information," included a wealth of detailed scientific data concerning the medicinal use of the waters in the town that offered the "sick and convalescent important and incomparable conditions for healing." The contrast with medical guides from the first half of the nineteenth century is striking. Supported by scientific studies of therapeutic efficacy, the assertions made were a far cry from the panacea claims nearly ubiquitous as late as the 1850s. Only seven concrete indications are listed with suggestions regarding how the waters were effectively applied by spa balneologists.[36] This represented a real, not simply a cosmetic change. Balneologists had in fact narrowed their scope and honed their methods much in accordance with the agenda set out in the 1850s.

The promotional efforts undertaken in Baden-Baden were similar to those of other spas. Archival records show that Heiligenthal's advertisement, spurred by his discovery of the Wiesbaden example, was not an isolated occurrence; frequently, Baden-Baden responded to initiatives taken in

[34] Emanuel Hirsch, *Wie soll der Kranke im Kurorte Leben. Ärztliche Ratschläge.* (Berlin: Alfred Pulvermacher & Co. medizin. Verlag, 1909), 10.
[35] Hans-Ulrich Wehler, *Deutsche Gesellschaftsgeschichte* (Munich: C.H. Beck, 1995) 3: 735.
[36] *Baden-Baden, Seine Kurmittel und Thermen*, 1909, in StA BB 20-13-8.

other spas.[37] It worked the other way, too. Wiesbaden produced a medical festschrift celebrating its own new Kaiser Friedrich Bad, which included high-resolution illustrations of the equipment.[38] Newspapers ran so-called "correspondence reports" not only from Baden-Baden, which many mistook for objective news stories. In 1913, a Berlin biweekly, the Berlin *Börsenkurier*, proposed to run, but not for free, a special section on Baden-Baden in a series on spas that included Kissingen, Ems, and Wiesbaden. The Cure Committee approved funding for the project, which alongside entertaining pieces, would also highlight the latest medical studies. [39] General guidebooks followed the same pattern as those for Baden-Baden, listing all the therapies available, and often including the names and addresses of practicing physicians, but omitting instructions on the use of the waters.

Spa advertising in the last decades of the nineteenth century continued to utilize forms it had since early in the century, but assumed a substantially different character. Promotion to the general public was expanded to reach a larger, national audience. These efforts excluded the kind of information denounced by balneologists in the 1850s as inappropriate, even dangerous. After about 1870, potential patients were no longer privy to knowledge that would enable them to bypass spa physicians and treat themselves. Even publications directed toward referring physicians were much more reticent about techniques, offering scientific explanations of how and why therapies were effective, yet remaining silent about the manner in which these were conducted. This was in stark contrast to the medical discourse presented in medical guides in previous decades. The trend away from *Wasserheilkunde*, tainted with the legacy of Romanticism and Galenic humoral pathology, is evident; authors were loath to even mention the word. The list of hydrotherapeutic indications grew more precise, as any sort of magical notions or panacea claims vanished from the pages of the guides. Instead, the authors rested their assertions of therapeutic efficacy on concrete, scientific studies, embracing the movement toward the scientific discipline of balneology pioneered in the 1850s and 1860s. This meant expert knowledge. The initiates in the

[37] See StA BB 20-13-8, StA BB 20-17-155 "Curörtliche Verhältnisse," Correspondence between Franz Heiligenthal and the Cure Committee, May, 1877.
[38] F. Blumenfeld, H. Fresenius, R. Friedlaender et al., *Ärztliche Festschrift zur Eröffnung des Städtischen Kaiser Friedrich Bades in Wiesbaden* (Wiesbaden: J.F. Bergmann, 1913).
[39] Sta BB 20-13-12, "Herausgabe des Neuen Prospectes, 1897." Report from the Verkehrsverein to the *Cur Comité*, March 10, 1913.

mysteries of the field were not just medical doctors in general, but had become specialists.

How successful these promotional efforts would turn out to be was, of course, an open question at the beginning of the campaign. In 1872, no one in Baden-Baden could be sure of what the future would hold. The insistent focus on curing, long the emphasis in other spas, was a new strategy for Baden-Baden. The spa's survival became all the more perilous in the aftermath of the Franco-Prussian War, when the French, who had constituted up to one third of all the town's visitors prior to 1870, now largely boycotted the German resort, and on both sides of the border bathers adopted "thermal nationalism," patronizing spas at home.[40] The Cure Committee and local businessmen had to wonder if recasting Baden-Baden's images as first and foremost a place of curing would attract enough visitors to save their town from decline.

By 1886, after some fluctuations, the answer could no longer be in doubt. In a speech given at a banquet held in Baden-Baden on April 7, the president of the Upper Chamber of the parliament, August Lamey, toasted the success of the spa's efforts to rejuvenate itself. As the *Badeblatt* reported the following day:

> President Lamey responded … A town that grew so quickly and strongly [KW:. Baden-Baden] must have a strong attractive power … The casino has vanished and will soon be forgotten. Baden has overcome the crisis in exemplary fashion; in the healing baths a replacement has been found … Baden's reputation is growing constantly, its blossoming one that will last.[41]

Visitor statistics confirm that the Badenese politician's words were not simply glib remarks made on a festive occasion. Over fifty-six thousand patrons sought out Baden-Baden in 1868, over thirteen thousand of whom were from France.[42] The first year without the casino, 1873, only thirty-eight thousand visitors came, meaning that not only the French stayed away. The following years of economic depression were not particularly rosy for the resort-town, with an average of some forty thousand annually. By 1884, however, steady growth in the number of visitors had returned, and in 1886, when Lamey celebrated success, the pre-1870 level had been

[40] Mackaman, *Leisure Settings*, 65.

[41] Article in the *Badener Wochenblatt* (April 8, 1886): 361-62. The article was clipped and preserved in the archives, StA BB 20-17-155.

[42] Frech, *Der Kurort Baden-Baden*, 37.

reached again.[43] By 1898, Baden-Baden had far surpassed its past numbers, hosting 61,347 visitors.[44]

What was the reason behind this growth? Did pleasure seekers simply return to familiar environs once economic prosperity allowed them again to take a vacation? Evidence suggests that the promotion formula stressing medical treatment was in fact effective. The new Friedrichsbad was an unmitigated success, so popular that it soon was unable to accommodate all those who wished to take advantage of its amenities. A second monumental bathhouse exclusively for women, the Kaiserin-Augusta Bad, was dedicated in 1893, with the Friedrichsbad continuing to host the men. Even in the less prosperous years of the late 1870s and early 1880s, an ever-increasing number of baths were administered in the Friedrichsbad, from just over thirty thousand in 1878, to 55,846 in 1884. It was not the case, as one might suspect, that visitors simply flocked to the sparkling new bathhouse. Private facilities continued to administer nearly half of the total number of baths given, which rose from 66,647 in 1878 to 102,349 in 1884.[45] The number of visitors in these years increased by around twenty percent; the number of baths, however, by over fifty percent.

To what extent the introduction of health insurance in 1883 contributed to this development is difficult to ascertain. The insurance laws gave academic physicians additional clout in their attempts to corner the market,[46] but the evidence suggests its effect in the spa world was not substantial, a distinct and curious feature. There was, in fact, an increase in the number of visitors between 1882 and 1884, but this upward trend had already begun before the spike in the numbers which probably had little to do with the introduction of health insurance payments. To be sure, the access provided by health insurance schemes did enable many to take advantage of professional medical care. Health insurance legislation, however, expanded on an already existing basis, and at first only covered a

[43] Loeser, *Geschichte der Stadt Baden*, 429.

[44] *Deutschlands Heilquellen und Bäder. Herausgegeben vom Kaiserlichen Gesundheits-Amt zu Berlin* (Berlin: Oswald Seehagen's Verlag (Martin Hoefer), 1900), 21.

[45] StA BB 20-17-155, "Tabellarische Uebersicht über die Bäderabgabe in den Großherzoglichen und Privatbadeanstalten in den Jahren 1878 bis mit 1884."

[46] Claudia Huerkamp, "Die preußisch-deutsche Ärzteschaft als Teil des Bildungsbürgertums" in Werner Conze and Jürgen Kocka, eds., *Bildungsbürgertum im 19. Jahrhundert. Teil 1, Bildungssystem und Professionalisierung im internationalen Vergleichen* (Stuttgart: Klett-Cotta, 1985), 379 ff.

relatively small number of workers. It expanded slowly until by 1900, a large segment of the German population could benefit from payments.[47]

The introduction and expansion of health insurance plans, however, did not radically change the curing landscape in spas like Baden-Baden. Working class and *Mittelstand* beneficiaries of the *Krankenkassen* who did find their way to Baden-Baden were shunted off into separate facilities, much as the poor had been segregated into the poor bath in earlier decades. The finer establishments, as well as stubbornly independent private practitioners, charged fees far higher than could be defrayed by insurance benefits. Separate facilities existed to provide care for such "insurance-only" patients, that at the same protected the exclusivity of the upscale establishments, long the preserves of the wealthy.

The legacy of the poor bath or *Armenbad* continued in a new form in the world of social insurance. Two institutions admitted insurance patients: the city hospital and the *Landesbad* or state bath. The city hospital, first constructed in 1860, underwent a substantial expansion in the 1880s to accommodate the new influx of patients of moderate means. The hospital and the old *Armenbad* could not offer sufficient space to meet demand, and so a replacement was necessary. The solution lay in a new *Landesbad* specifically designed to accept patients whose therapy was financed by the *Krankenkassen.* Conceived in the mid-1880s, construction began in 1887, and the new *Landesbad* entered into service in 1890. While in theory the *Landesbad* was open to all willing to pay for a stay, and offered more expensive rooms for those able to do so, most patients staying at these facilities opted for the simplest accommodation, and were supported by insurance payments. Few people who paid their own way chose to stay in the public facility.[48]

The *Landesbad*, which charged between 1-2 marks daily for the insured and 2.50 –3 marks daily for those paying their own way, was less than half the price of a mid-range hotel, and included more services.[49] For many, especially those likely to be insured, private accommodation was prohibitively expensive. A stay in a mid-range hotel would set a guest back at least five and as much as twelve marks a day, not including baths or any medical treatment. Even a "private eye clinic for persons of limited means" [*Privat Augenheil-Anstalt mit Vereinsaugenklinik für Unbemittelte*] which in 1890 treated 1,133 patients, 237 of whom were inpatients,

---

[47] Ute Frevert, "Professional Medicine and the Working Classes in Imperial Germany," in *Journal of Contemporary History* 20, no. 4 (October 1984): 637-658.

[48] Loeser, *Geschichte der Stadt Baden*, 369.

[49] Loeser, *Geschichte der Stadt Baden*, 369.

charged between 3.50 and five marks daily. This was the bargain rate: a more typical price was that charged for the presumably more exclusive private section, between eight and twenty five marks daily.[50] Some context is necessary to make sense of these figures. In 1892, 70.27 percent of the German population had an income under 900 marks annually.[51] The cost of a fourteen-day stay in a private clinic (when a proper cure was thought to take between fourteen and twenty-one days), at least 112 and more likely 350 marks, was clearly well out of reach of a large segment of the population, namely those most likely to be covered by health insurance. Clearly, private sanatoria were the domain of patients who paid for treatment themselves.

The force of prices was perhaps most instrumental in directing the lower classes into public facilities removed from the more elegant private hotels and sanatoria. The Friedrichsbad was open to *Insassen* (literally, inmates) of the *Landesbad* only during the least desirable hours in the afternoon (regarded as therapeutically inferior) when presumably the wealthy (who paid a premium admission price) would not be inconvenienced. Other matters of policy, too, served to show public patients their place, as a small incident that took place in the local tourist office illustrates. In 1907, one J. Bossert wrote to the city council with a complaint. The man went with two acquaintances to the city information office to request a copy of the Baden-Baden brochure. The clerk working in the office, one Mr. Heidecke, asked if the gentlemen were staying in the *Landesbad.* Two were, and they were not given the brochure, while the third man, not from the *Landesbad*, was given a copy. An argument ensued, in which the gentlemen were informed, an allegation later denied by Mr. Heidecke, that the city had already provided many special advantages and discounts for "inmates" of the *Landesbad*, and they should not make unreasonable demands. The three men, schoolteachers by profession, left the office, offended. The director of the City Information Office responded to the city council that this policy, "often leading to false impressions ... hardly involved disrespect to inmates of the *Landesbad*," yet nevertheless needed to be upheld, as to do otherwise would "in no way resonate with the propagandistic [*propagandistisch*] tendencies that we

---

[50] StA BB 26-29-173, "Verkehrswesen: Prospekt von BB, 1906." Advertising brochure from 1906 listing the hotels, inns and sanatoria in Baden-Baden, including prices.
[51] Hajo Holborn, *A History of Modern Germany, 1840-1945* (Princeton, NJ: Princeton University Press, Paperback Edition, 1982), 389-90.

have had to follow in the interest of our spa."[52] The episode ended with a decision by the mayor to send one hundred copies of the brochure to the *Landesbad*, to reduce tensions, and, presumably to preempt inmate visits to the information office.

The paying customers of Baden-Baden, solidly middle- and upper-class patrons, continued to dominate the spa. In stark contrast with the casino days of the 1850s, however, the emphasis on curing had borne fruit by the 1880s, and greater numbers of guests arrived for the treatment of ailments. Like their less well-off counterparts, more affluent visitors came largely to take the waters, and in doing so, sought medical counsel. As has been argued for Bad Ems during the last decades of the nineteenth century, "with the preponderance of the sick among the visitors … the majority of spa guests consulted a physician."[53]

This claim, based on physicians' practice records, may be somewhat overstated, for those seeking amusement and relaxation remained a significant part of the public. As Theodor Fontane, a habitué of the spas, wrote after a most uncomfortable stay in Silesia, "one finds this combination of air and light and freshness, and of comfort and pleasure only in the larger spas, of which Germany, thank God, has so many: Interlaken, Regaz, Baden-Baden, Wiesbaden, Kissingen, Karlsbad, that one can seek out, even without being a patient. I in the end became devoted entirely to these."[54] Ideally, of course, a sojourn in a spring town would combine both leisure and curing. Pleasure certainly did not disappear under the watchful eye of a physician. Guests expected a level of comfort, and offering such provided exclusivity and added appeal. Friedrich Nietzsche, a man not noted for flattery, took a cold-water cure in Baden-Baden from March 2 to April 4, 1878 and felt called upon to state that the comfort in his hotel and in the bathhouse "was beyond all praise!"[55]

---

[52] StA BB 26-29-173. Letter from the Tourist Office, October 8, 1907, in response to a letter of complaint from J. Bossert to the City Council of Baden-Baden, October 3, 1907.

[53] Sommer, *Zur Kur Nach Ems. Ein Beitrag zur Geschichte der Baderise von 1830 bis 1914*. Geschichtliche Landeskunde, Bd. 48, (Franz Steiner Verlag, Stuttgart, 1999), 608.

[54] Theodor Fontane, "Die Sommerfrischen," in: *Von Zwanzig bis Dreissig. Autobiographisches Nebst anderen selbstbiographischen Zeugnissen.* [Originally published 1898] in *Theodor Fontane, Sämtliche Werke*, Kurt Schreinert and Jutta Neuendorff-Fürstenau, eds. (Munich: Nymphenburger Verlagshandlung, 1967), 25: 394-95. For a brief discussion of Fontane's preference for Kissingen and Karlsbad, see Helmuth Nürnberger, *Fontanes Welt* (Berlin: Siedler, 1997), 383.

[55] Haebler, *Geschichte der Stadt und des Kurortes*, 2: 142.

Medical treatment, not pleasure-seeking, also took pride of place in humorous accounts of spa life. Tongue-in-cheek, one observer described the prevailing "spa fever" as "nothing more than a stage in the general illness."[56] Everyone was ill and everything pathological, and so spending summers in a spa was only logical. For every malady there was a spa, heralded by advertising that promised its cure. Consequently, anyone who was respectable might be expected to have a genteel illness or "condition" that absolutely required a visit to the spa for the summer season. Illness, real or imagined, suffered or feared, remained a strong motivation for guests. A 1900 guide to manners offered a more complete picture. "Part of the spa guests come in order to seek and find restoration of their health under the direction of a physician … [others] to introduce some distraction into the routine of their lives … and frequently spa visits are even undertaken in the hope of assisting adolescent daughters to a future."[57] Discernible here is the triad of motives for a spa visit that dated back to the beginning of the nineteenth century: health, diversion, or the hope of easy romance. Yet within this triad, a source of tension throughout the history of the spa, the pursuit of health under the direction of a physician had gained preponderance over the other two.

Despite the enduring presence of travelers for pleasure, the growth of private sanatoria demonstrate that a growing number of visitors came to Baden-Baden in order to submit to a medical regimen. Dr. Hoffmann's private ophthalmological clinic was opened in 1875; by 1900, there were at least six such private sanatoria, and by 1905, eleven.[58] Nor was this development unique to Baden-Baden. Spurred in part by the growth of railroads, private sanatoria sprang up in spas across German-speaking Europe throughout the last decades of the nineteenth century.[59] The types of maladies treated in these clinics varied, ranging from nervous disorders, including the widespread and diffuse diagnosis of neurasthenia, to substance abuse, tuberculosis, and convalescence from trauma and other

---

[56] Adolf Löwenstein, "Badekuren," in: *Humor in der Medizin* (Berlin: Erwin Staude, 1875), 81.
[57] Franz Ebhardt, *Der Gute Ton in allen Lebenslagen* (Leipzig and Berlin: Verlag von Julius Klinkhardt, 1900), 582-583.
[58] See Baumgärtner, et al. *Baden-Baden und seine Kurmittel*, 141; *Deutschlands Heilquellen und Bäder*, 21; H. Oefflinger, *Die Kurorte und Heilquellen des Grossherzogtums Baden für Aerzte und Heilbedürftige* (Baden-Baden, Sommermeyer, 1905), 20.
[59] Edward Shorter, "Private Clinics in Central Europe, 1850-1933," *Social History of Medicine* 3, no. 2 (1990): 159-195.

acute ailments.[60] Treatment tended to be holistic in nature, with therapy supplementing use of mineral waters and with prescribed diet, exercise, and rest. Patients voluntarily submitted themselves to a curative regimen under the direct supervision of a physician and paid for the privilege. The success of these sanatoria in spas across Germany underscores the change in the nature of a spa visit. Earlier in the century, leisure was often only supplemented by curing; by the 1890s curing, which had grown increasingly elaborate, had now assumed the unquestionably dominant position. Doctors were seeing the fruits of their efforts, and had succeeded in gaining a position of authority with their patients in the spa.

Private water institutes [*Wasserheilanstalten*] tended incresasingly to treat psychiatric disorders. That they constituted a large part of patients in spas and balneological sanatoria was widely-known among doctors, but this fact was hushed and kept from the public.[61] To a great degree, clinics offering psychotherapy were located in spas, and for patients with sufficient means and for whom admission to a psychiatric hospital carried too much of a stigma, taking a private cure at a spa was a viable way to seek therapy, and one that preserved patient dignity.

Among the various ailments frequently treated in private clinics, the most frequent single condition was neurasthenia, or nervousness, thought to arise from nervous irritation.[62] Neurasthenia defied clear, concrete diagnosis or treatment, perhaps, because it could manifest itself with a broad range of symptoms, including agitation, gastrointestinal complaints,

---

[60] Edward Shorter, "Private Clinics in Central Europe, 1850-1933," 172.

[61] Shorter, "Private Clinics in Central Europe, 1850-1933," 170.

[62] Neurasthenia was first identified by a New York physician, George M. Beard, in 1880, and quickly 'spread' to Germany, where it became a widely diagnosed condition and part of popular discourse outside the control of medicine. Precisely what the widespread 'cultural disease' neurasthenia was remains a subject of some debate, with some scholars regarding the ailment as a cultural phenomenon, others as a genuine epidemic of the late nineteenth century, others still as simply a general diagnosis or even a euphemism for various psychosomatic disorders. An in-depth discussion of this issue is well beyond the scope of this study, but has received detailed scholarly treatment in a recent monograph. See Joachim Radkau, *Das Zeitalter der Nervösität. Deutschland zwischen Bismarck und Hitler* (Munich: Propyläen, 2000). See also Wolfgang U. Eckhart, "Die wachsende Nervösität underer Zeit.' Medizin und Kultur um 1900 am Beispiel einer Modekrankheit." in G. Hübinger, R. v. Bruch, F.W. Graf, eds., *Kultur und Kulturwissenschaften um 1900. Vol. II, Idealismus und Positivismus* (Stuttgart: Steiner Verlag, 1997), 207-226; Martina Kessel, *Langeweile. Zum Umgang mit Zeit und Gefühlen in Deutschland vom späten 18. bis zum frühen 20. Jahrhundert* (Göttingen: Wallstein, 2001).

sexual dysfunction (hyper- or hypoactivity), lethargy, heart palpatations and so on. Spreading across Germany in epidemic proportions after 1880, this diffusely-described and frequently diagnosed illness was perfectly suited for spa treatment, where nature-based therapies and a peaceful atmosphere could at least serve as a palliative, if not a cure.

It has been argued that neurasthenia was devised by the medical community in order to strengthen its hold over the population and to increase its authority by finding a condition from which millions suffered either chronically or intermittently. Arising perhaps out of medical practice, and almost certainly linked with the stress of life in the modern technological world and with sexual repression, neurasthenia, however, was not necessarily in the interests of a specializing medical-scientific establishment. The nebulous origin and diagnosis of neurasthenia ran counter to the trend toward medical specialization, and was "more compatible with natural medicine than with scientific medicine."[63] These "natural healers," who most often were not academic physicians, treated neurasthenia as a disease of civilization, arising from the problems of life in modern society, and advocated a return to nature. Their efforts were no less effective apparently than those of academic medicine. Paul Möbius, the physician who perhaps more than any other helped spread the word about neurasthenia, himself conceded that with nervous patients, "quacks had no less success than scientifically respectable physicians."[64] For this malady at least, laboratory-based scientific medicine of the kind pioneered in the 1850s and 1860s could not offer significantly better results. This certainly did not help the cause of scientific medicine.

It was in part a result of neurasthenia that the natural therapy movement and other alternative medical movements such as homeopathy, were reinvigorated in the last decades of the nineteenth century. Many, including a significant number of physicians, felt that compartmentalized laboratory medicine was insufficient to treat every illness, as neurasthenia made clear. Alternative medicine's comeback was not only a response to the relative inefficacy of academic medicine in treatment of widespread ailments, but represented also broad resistance to the hegemonic efforts of

---

[63] Radkau, *Das Zeitalter der Nervösität*, 91.

[64] Paul Julius Möbius, cited in Radkau, *Das Zeitalter der Nervösität*, 91. Möbius was an academic physician and prolific medical writer. One of his most interesting works, perhaps, which among other things argued "scientifically" why women were not suited for the medical profession, *Über den physiologischen Schwachsinn des Weibes* (Halle: 1900) ran through at least ten editions by 1912, and was recently reprinted in a facsimile edition (Munich: Matthes & Seitz, 1990), as an item of historical interest.

academically-trained physicians. Increasingly specialized after 1870, they laid claim to a monopoly on genuine medical knowledge that had the effect of placing patients into a subordinate role. As one participant at the 1878 convention of German Natural Scientists and Physicians blithely asserted: "The gospel of the scientific method has long been preached to us physicians. And whosoever among physicians does not confess allegiance to this gospel, he no longer deserves, as I dare openly say, the title of a physician."[65]

In the end, university medicine came to be regarded as mainstream medicine, with schools of thought such as natural healing, homeopathy, and balneology regarded as alternative medicine. In the late nineteenth century, and into the twentieth, this triumphal march of laboratory medicine appeared far from inevitable, however. The struggle was not simply one between modernist progressive physicians versus backward-looking critics, but rather hinged on a difference in vision of how to approach healing in the modern industrial world. Academic medicine based its claims on bacteriology, physiology, and biochemistry, asserting an essentially, if recognizably limited, positivistic approach. Disease could be fully understood, quantified, and treated once the physiological causes were identified.[66]

Natural healers worked from a different set of premises regarding health and illness, one reminiscent of Romantic medicine, which integrated the person-patient with nature.[67] Natural therapy presented a considerable threat to scientific, allopathic medicine, because it enjoyed broad popularity from a variety of people and for diverse reasons. Bismarck was sympathetic, as were his political enemies, the Social Democrats. Even some officials in the health insurance system expressed an interest in alternative medicine as a way of combating the rising costs of scientific medicine. By 1914, some 900 voluntary associations for natural healing had nearly 200,000 members, making the movement a strong challenger to the claims of exclusivity made by mainstream

---

[65] Proceedings of the 1878 Versammlung Deutscher Naturforscher und Ärzte, Kassel, excerpted in Robert Jütte, *Geschichte der alternativen Medizin* (Munich: Beck, 1996), 28.

[66] See Eckhart, *Geschichte der Medizin*, Chapter 9, 249-318, especially 309-313.

[67] Martin Dinges, "Einleitung," in Martin Dinges, ed., *Medizinkritische Bewegungen im Deutschen Reich (ca. 1870–ca. 1933)*, MedGG Beihefte 9 (Stuttgart: Steiner Verlag, 1996), 16-17.

professional medicine.[68] As outsiders, they opposed the conventions of what by this time had to be considered established experimental allopathic medicine.

The response of academic physicians to the challenge of the natural healers only served to sharpen the conflict, playing into the hands of the enemy. Physicians' own confidence in the superiority of their brand of scientific medicine led many, including the influential Berlin Medical Society, to advocate the passage of a general "*Kurierfreiheit*" (freedom of practice) statute in 1869.[69] Under this legislation, which applied to the German Reich as a whole in 1871, practitioners without academic degrees were allowed to treat patients, for only the title of physician (*Arzt*) was regulated. Physicians believed that open competition with scientific academic medicine would inevitably discredit non-academic quacks, and serve better to eliminate them for good than any prohibition. The result was the reverse of what physicians had expected: rather than eliminating such alternative practitioners, the door was open wide to them, and their numbers mushroomed as people sought alternatives to academic medicine. In attempting to quash the competition, academic physicians, in fact, provided favorable conditions in which their rivals could thrive.

One such practitioner who gained considerable fame and reputation in the late nineteenth century was Sebastian Kneipp, a lay-healer and Roman Catholic priest, who adapted mostly existing knowledge of cold-water therapy in his *Wasserheilanstalt*, opened in 1881 in the Bavarian village of Wörishofen. His popularity soared after publication of his manual, *Meine Wasserkur* in 1886, which ran through fifty editions in only eight years.[70] Kneipp's method, as the sales of his book suggest, spread quickly across Germany, with hundreds of large and small *Wasserheilanstalten* practicing the Kneipp method by the turn of the century.[71]

---

[68] Cornelia Regin, "Zwischen Angriff und Abwehr. Die Naturheilbewegung als medizinkritische Öffentlichkeit im Deutschen Kaiserreich." in Dinges, *Medizinkritische Bewegungen*, 39. See also Radkau, *Das Zeitalter der Nervösität*, 92.

[69] Claudia Huerkamp, "Ärzte und Professionalisierung in Deutschland. Überlegungen zum Wandel des Arztberufs im 19. Jahrhundert." in *Geschichte und Gesellschaft* 6, no. 1 (1980): 365; see also Charles E. McClelland, "Modern German Doctors: A Failure of Professionalization?" in Manfred Berg and Geoffrey Cocks, eds., *Medicine and Modernity: Public Health and Medical Care in Nineteenth- and Twentieth-Century Germany* (Washington, DC: German Historical Institute and Cambridge University Press, 1996), 86.

[70] Horst Prignitz, *Wasserkur und Badelust: Eine Badereise in die Vergangenheit* (Leipzig: Koehler & Amelang, 1986), 191.

[71] Prignitz, *Wasserkur und Badelust*, 193.

Kneipp, like his predecessor Priessnitz, had no medical training and, as supposedly developed his therapy after insights gained by self-experimentation. Unlike Priessnitz, however, Kneipp's method did not disappear after his death in 1897. To be sure, the popularity of natural healing helped Kneipp therapy to survive beyond its founder's death, but in part it survived thanks to spa physicians. In contrast to their rejection of Priessnitz in the 1850s, many spa physicians attempted to co-opt Kneipp, using his methods under the auspices of "proper scientific method and supervision." Significantly, each of the Kneipp *Wasserheilanstalten* in 1900 soon stood under the direction of an academic physician.[72] The Association of Kneipp Physicians [*Kneippärztebund*] was founded in 1894 to promote the method, secure its reputation in the scientific community, and to exercise control over it. In this last regard, however, the Association was a failure, in that Kneipp's teachings were spread and to a large extent taken over not by scientific-medical associations, but by lay organizations.[73] Although Kneipp therapy continued to attract some physicians, once it became clear that it could not be controlled by the academically trained establishment, the efforts of the Association to integrate it into mainstream medicine, even mainstream spa medicine, were not a striking success, and the movement remained in large part one advanced by laymen, not medical professionals.

The growth of such lay associations was particularly threatening to spa physicians. Allopathic physicians could dismiss approaches such as Kneipp therapy as unscientific and ineffective, even harmful. Balneologists could ill-afford take such a position, in that their own practice was not only similar, but in part had adopted Priessnitz' and Kneipp's techniques. Among skeptics, lay approaches to hydrotherapy therefore undermined spa physicians' claims to legitimacy as serious scientific practitioners, and at the same time undermined the confidence of the faithful in their unrivaled possession of specialist expertise. In order to "force out the influence of laymen,"[74] the movement had to be co-opted and then embossed with the stamp of science. A careful balance between assertion of authority and acceptance of outsiders' popular innovations had to be found. The Baden-Baden spa physician Corval wrote with characteristic ambivalence in 1886 that Priessnitz' "merit should not be underestimated; he at any rate invented cold-water therapy and developed an application that we mostly use today, after eliminating certain excesses, and understandably with

[72] Prignitz, *Wasserkur und Badelust*, 193.

[73] Gerhard Hüfner, *Die wissenschaftlichen Vereinigungen im deutschen Heilbäderwesen 1878-1994* (Gütersloh: Flottmann Verlag, 1994), 53.

[74] Radkau, *Das Zeitalter der Nervösität*, 92.

progressively more scientific developments…"[75] Not to give the wrong impression, however, Corval also lambasted Priessnitz for his lack of scientific method which had dangerous consequences. Science, in the hands of a proper physician, had rendered Priessnitz' method safe and effective.

Glib statements that lay practices had been rendered scientific in the hands of experts were hardly sufficient to secure professional standing, however, and needed to be supported by more concrete efforts. The key, in addition to promotion, lay in organization. In an environment in which professional societies dedicated to the promotion of scientific, academic medicine were forming, it was particularly important for spa physicians, still struggling for recognition from their colleagues at universities, to establish their own scientific standing and to reduce the impact of laymen in their field of hydrotherapy. Reviving the efforts begun by Ludwig Spengler in the 1850s, balneologists in 1878 attempted to establish a balneological section of the influential Congress of Natural Researchers and Physicians. Their efforts failed. Undeterred, they founded such a section within the less prestigious but evidently more accommodating Society for Therapeutics [*Gesellschaft für Heilkunde*] in October 1878, which was transformed into the Balneological Society [*Balneologische Gesellschaft*] in 1889. These societies sought to integrate balneology and climatology, the core disciplines of spa medicine, into mainstream university medicine.

Georg Thilenius, a third-generation *Badearzt* and a National Liberal parliamentarian in the Prussian parliament and for Wiesbaden in the Reichstag, commented on the 1878 failure. Trying perhaps to make the best of a bad situation, he expounded in the *Deutsche Medizinische Wochenschrift* on the purpose and position of the society:

> Never will I be able to understand the discipline of mineral spring therapy as anything but a branch of the *material medica*, as a discipline intimately linked with the practice of the art of medicine. … Balneotherapy can only properly flourish if its practitioners remain in lively interaction with other practicing physicians. On the other hand, no one will wish to deny that the peculiar nature of balneotherapy affords it a particular position among therapeutic approaches and forces its practitioners to treat it as a medical specialty.[76]

---

[75] Dr. v. Corval, "Hydrotherapie" in Baumgärtner, et al., *Baden-Baden und seine Kurmittel*, 106.

[76] Georg Thileneus, *Deutsche Medizinische Wochenschrift*, 5 (1879), 136, cited in Hüfner, *Die wissenschaftlichen Vereinigungen im deutschen Heilbäderwesen*, 22.

In his keynote address at the 1879 conference of the Society for Therapeutics in Berlin, Thilenius made his point even more directly:

> I assume I am assured of your agreement when I say that–and let us admit it openly–we can reshape our relations with the rest of the medical world, that are much in need of improvement, if we recognize the solidarity of our interests.[77]

The purpose, then, of organization was to improve interaction with the remainder of the medical community. This did not mean just friendly collegial relations, good will, and warm feelings, but recognition and respect. The situation had not improved much from that of the 1850s, when Spengler launched his efforts to establish the scientific credibility of the field; in many ways it had grown more critical. With the emergence of alternative medicine, which in part was defined as such by criticism from the growing academic medical establishment, balneologists essentially faced the choice of joining the dissenters or struggling to remain part of that medical establishment.

The statutes and publications of balneological professional associations make clear which path had been chosen. The 1889 founding statute of the Balneological Society underscored the need for the "advancement of scientific balneology with all [its] strength [and] to promote collegial relations between all balneologists and to practical physicians."[78] The All German Association of Mineral Baths [*Allgemeiner Deutscher Bäderverband*] committed to a similar purpose at its founding in 1892, devoting itself to the promotion of spas and acting as a "constant liaison with the representatives of the entire field of scientific medicine and the natural sciences."[79] The pages of the *Medizinische Woche*, the official organ of the Conference of Black Forest Spas the Association of North Sea Baths and the Association of Baltic Spa Physicians launched in 1900 are filled with reports from the world of academic medicine, polemics for the

---

[77] Thilenius, Keynote address to the *Gesellschaft für Heilkunde* in Berlin, January 25, 1879, excerpted in Hüfner, *Die wissenschaftlichen Vereinigungen im deutschen Heilbäderwesen*, 48.

[78] Paragraph 2 of the founding statutes of the Balenologische Gesellschaft, reproduced in Hüfner, *Die wissenschaftlichen Vereinigungen im deutschen Heilbäderwesen*, 25.

[79] Paragraph 2 of the founding statutes of the Allgemeiner Deutscher Bäderverband, founded April 23, 1892, reproduced in Hüfner, *Die Deutschen Bäderverbände, 1892-1992. Chronik der Verbandsarbeit* (Gütersloh: Flöttmann Verlag, 1992), 39-45.

advancement of balneology as a full member of the community of medical fields.

A related and recurrent theme in the issues of the *Medizinische Woche* was the struggle against quackery, in other words, lay practitioners and alternative medicine. An article by Ernst Thessing attacked the full range of quacks, from non-licensed practitioners, opponents of immunization, midwives, and went on to include individuals attempting to treat themselves. A legislative reversal of the *Kurierfreiheit*, Thessing asserted, would be ineffective, as this would not combat the root of the problem, which ultimately resided in a stubbornly skeptical segment of the population. Thessing was not uncritical of academic medicine, and admitted that unlicensed lay practitioners may have been able to achieve some material and therapeutic successes. This he ascribed to their ability to address the whole patient, including his or her psychological and emotional needs, an area which he found lacking in conventional physicians. The thrust of the argument, however, was that clinicians had to combine the holistic view of the patient offered by "quacks" in order to convince even skeptics of the superiority of academic medicine. Education of both patients and physicians was they key to eradicating the problem of lay practitioners.

Others, however, were not so reasonable. Regretting the miscalculation of the *Kurierfreiheit*, physicians' professional associations sought unsuccessfully to reverse it.[80] On the local level, too, spa administrations took action to suppress lay practitioners within their jurisdiction, making use of police powers to harass unlicensed competitors with the hope of at least driving them out of town. The well-documented case in Baden-Baden of the conflict between the Cure Committee and just such a lay practitioner, Rudolf Blitz, is illustrative of the manner in which established spa physicians could defend their turf.

Blitz first came to Baden-Baden in 1903 in order to establish a branch of the "Society for the Prevention of Illness in the Human Race," of which he was the general superintendent. The purpose of this society, according to its charter and publications, was "the prevention of all illnesses and to make possible for each individual a healthy existence, to discover all causes of illness in humanity, and to educate the populace through all fields of natural philosophy, not medicine."[81] Moreover, the statutes of the society were directly antagonistic toward academic medicine, stating

---

[80] Huerkamp, "Die preußisch-deutsche Ärzteschaft," 379.

[81] GLAKa 339/1338, "Medizinalwesen, Nichtapprobierte Heilpersonal," Brochure of the Gesellschaft zur Vorbeugung der Krankheit in der menschlichen Rasse, 1903.

directly that the new science advocated by the society had as its express purpose a correction of academic medicine's errors:

> The object of the results of the new science [is] to resolve the existing errors in the science of medicine, to halt its mistaken methods and inadequate prescriptions, as these are more inclined to increase the suffering in humanity than to reduce it.[82]

From the outset, officials in Baden-Baden were highly suspicious of Blitz. The day he registered with the police (a standard procedure), medical authorities notified the *Bezirksamt* and questioned his legitimacy. Soon afterward, a copy of Blitz' police record was requested from Berlin, which returned perfectly clean. Nevertheless, police agents were assigned to place him under surveillance; the regular reports from their investigations exposed no suspicious activity.

Blitz, like many medical men in spas, licensed doctors and non-licensed practitioners alike, spent the summer season in Baden-Baden and the winter in Nice. His résumé, which the *Bezirksamt* had in its files, as well as the brochure of the society, showed that Blitz had spent considerable time practicing in France and in Philadelphia, where he had supposedly gained considerable recognition for his new methods.

Blitz called himself professor, a highly respected honorific, the misuse of which was prohibited. Officials investigated Blitz' past and discovered that while he indeed had a higher education, he had merely the qualifications of a *Volksschullehrer*, or middle-school teacher. In order to resolve the question as to where Blitz may have earned the title of professor, the investigation was widened to include inquiries by the Imperial German consulates in the cities where Blitz had lived in the past. None produced any evidence of any credentials, nor much information at all, despite his claims of fame abroad. The consulate in Philadelphia noted that in the United States, the title professor was meaningless unless attached to an academic institution, stating that here "any dance teacher can call himself 'Professor of Dancing.'"[83] A similar inquiry at the Consulate in Paris suggested that Blitz may have been using the title in the sense of the French *professeur*, which the consular report pointed out, could be used for any teacher.

---

[82] GLAKa 339/1338, Brochure of the Gesellschaft zur Vorbeugung der Krankheit in der menschlichen Rasse.

[83] GLAKa 339/1338, Letter from the Imperial German Consulate in Philadelphia to the Bezirksamt Baden, October 13, 1904.

Upon his return from Nice in the spring of 1904, Blitz was warned to cease and desist from making use of the title, which police agents had reported was posted on his doorbell. Blitz' disingenuous explanation was that he himself had no idea how the title may have appeared on his doorbell, supposing that perhaps it had been his landlord who had put it there. The sign was removed, but the matter did not end there. Police investigation of Blitz continued through 1904 and 1905, yet the worst it seemed he could be accused of, on the basis of hard evidence, that is, was an exaggeration of his claims.

What of Blitz' practice in Baden-Baden? Both the *Badearzt* and the *Bezirksarzt* were hostile toward him, as is evidenced by their hounding and the nature of their reports. Yet he enjoyed considerable success. At the first general meeting of his society in September 1904, well over one hundred persons were present to hear him speak, including, according to the police report, many respectable persons: teachers, officials, and notables. At this point, there were nearly sixty signed up members of the society in Baden-Baden, many of whom had donated considerable sums. Clearly, Blitz was popular, a fact that police surveillance of his patients could not deny. The "*Kurpfuscher*" [quack], one report grudgingly conceded, had achieved considerable successes in treating patients, particularly those who had suffered from chronic pain, rheumatism, and the like, or who had not been able to find relief from academic doctors, even university professors. It seems that in fact many people found relief from their suffering in his unorthodox therapy. While treatment was for members of the society, Blitz nevertheless was reported to have also treated gratis many of the local poor.

Nevertheless, the officials were not convinced, believing that "in spite of his clear therapeutic successes" he was a dubious person fixed on exploiting the public. They proceeded doggedly trying to build a case against him, monitoring his movements and statements. In the summer of 1905 charges were finally pressed against him. Despite the efforts of the Cure Committee in Baden-Baden to construct a case of fraud against him, the prosecutor's office closed the case when Blitz produced evidence of the legitimacy of his society and his method of collecting and using membership dues, as well as sworn testimony that he had not used any sort of deception to lure patients into his treatment, but rather that they had sought him out.[84]

---

[84] GLAKA 339/1338, Report of the Staatsanwaltschaft Karlsruhe, September 14, 1905.

Nevertheless, Blitz was prosecuted in the end, and lost on appeal. It was not fraud, but rather a minor infraction of a city ordinance which required practitioners without licenses to register a change of residence with the local district physician. Blitz had failed to do this and therefore was convicted. In 1906, he was sentenced to ten days imprisonment and a fine of 150 marks. This appears to have been the end of Blitz in Baden-Baden.

Certainly, Blitz was a suspicious figure. His use of the title "Professor" Blitz was almost certainly not one allowed by German law, and many of his other assertions about his qualifications were equally suspect. Be that as it may, he attracted a loyal following, as the intervention of satisfied patients on his behalf with the prosecutor's office demonstrated. This made Blitz precisely the kind of practitioner established physicians most feared: a convincing quack whose success undermined the authority of academically trained spa physicians by raising the specter of charlatanism for spa medicine as a whole.

Shady characters such as Blitz were not the only ones subject to police investigation. Medical doctors hailing from other parts of Germany or from abroad were subject to verification as well. So, for example, a supposed doctor and "American Dentist (from Rome)" advertising his services in 1880, A.H. Chamberlain, responded to the inquiry about his qualifications that he would leave Baden-Baden and not return. Others did not cave in so readily. In 1875, one Theodor Blondin tried to set up practice in Baden-Baden. His advertisements drew the attention of the authorities, since unlicensed (*nichtapprobiert*) individuals did not have the right to advertise. Blondin claimed to have been trained in France as a physician, but lacked a license to practice in Germany. For three years he struggled to gain recognition of his credentials, to no avail. Here was a case of a man that the authorities recognized was likely an academically trained physician, but being French-trained in the wake of the Franco-Prussian War certainly did not bolster his case.[85]

This did not mean that Germans went unchallenged. A physician setting up practice in Baden-Baden either would voluntarily register with the medical counselor (*Medizinalrat*) or would come under investigation after attempting to advertise. As a rule, however, physicians hailing from distant parts of Germany had little difficulty in securing their status. Occasionally, an investigation of a physician might be initiated pursuant to allegations about his character. In one such case in 1879, a police sergeant

[85] GLAKa 339/1446, "Medizinalwesen, Prüfung etc. der Ärzte, 1875-90." Correspondence of the Ministry of the Interior regarding the licensing petition of Dr. Theodor Blondin, January 16, 1875-October 30, 1878.

in neighboring Yburg wrote a letter regarding one Dr. Senff, who had recently established himself in Baden-Baden. The sergeant did not question the physician's qualifications, but rather suggested Senff was purely mercenary and refused to pay debts incurred for a lavish lifestyle, based on experiences he had with him in Lübeck and on his "entirely Jewish appearance."[86] That Senff may have been Jewish does not appear to have been an issue for anyone other than the police sergeant in Yburg; the police records noted some questions about Senff's character as an abrasive person, dismissed allegations that he might be an alcoholic, and that he left unpaid debts in Baden-Baden. The decision whether to investigate a particular physician or not seems to have been based on his origins. Foreign physicians were challenged *pro forma*, while those hailing from Germany were investigated only when there appeared to be substantive doubts about integrity. There is no evidence in the police records of any systematic investigation of Jewish physicians.

The attention devoted to the verification of physicians' credentials and surveillance of non-licensed practitioners testify that defending the integrity and reputation of the medical profession was a vital matter to spa authorities in Baden-Baden. Police officials and the Badenese Ministry of the Interior listened to the tips given by the spa administration, yet the members of the Cure Committee could not run roughshod over normal judicial procedures. If evidence did not substantiate a charge against a supposed charlatan, it was dismissed. Still, as the final outcome of Blitz' case suggests, determined authorities did in fact have at their disposal the resources and the latitude to eliminate a practitioner deemed a threat.

If physicians generally were interested in the removal of rivals from outside their guild –one of the hallmarks of successful professionalization– this was doubly so for balneologists who had to be concerned about their survival. Every questionable practitioner, every crackpot amateur, or even brilliant layman threatened the authority of balneology as a medical science. That is why efforts to discredit or eliminate non-licensed competitors could take on the character of a witch-hunt, as the Blitz case once again demonstrates. The credibility of spa medicine as serious science had to be defended against all threats, and it was better to err on the side of excessive vigilance than to show mercy.

How successful were these efforts? Did spa physicians succeed in the last decades of the nineteenth century in securing the status which they felt they deserved? If one examines one goal set in 1856 at the assembly of the

[86] GLAKa 339/1446, Letter from the *Amtshauptmann*, Yburg, to the Police Direction in Baden-Baden, July 15, 1879.

Balenological Society and cherished by many balneologists, namely the establishment of professorships in balneology at esteemed universities, the answer must be a negative one. Before 1914, there was not a single university institute in the field in all Germany.[87]

The lack of professorial chairs, however, did not mean that balneology and related fields were absent from the medical curriculum. From 1875-1914, University of Berlin showed a clear trend toward an increasing number of courses in balneology: from nine in the years 1875-1880, to twenty between 1895 and 1900, and thirty one in 1905-1910, with an additional number of courses offered in hydrotherapy and climatology.[88] Physicians, and professors in fields such as internal medicine or pathology often practiced balneology as well, and were members of the Balneological Society. Thilenius' successor as chair of the society was Oscar Liebrich, a professor of pharmacology in Berlin, and his successor, Ludwig Brieger, had written a habilitation in internal medicine also in Berlin.[89] Chairs of societies and university curricula can make only limited statements as to the spread and reputability of spa medicine, but they do suggest a degree of acceptance. Spa physicians, then, did succeed in establishing themselves as physicians proper, distinct from laymen such as Priessnitz and Kneipp, and distant from the likes of Blitz. Nevertheless, balneology remained a "stepchild of the scientific universities" in Germany and in other countries, acknowledged as a legitimate field, but lacking the prestige or position of such glamorous fields as bacteriology or surgery.[90] In trying to link the obvious nature-bound essence of their field with concrete science, balneology never entirely succeeded in shedding the air of natural philosophy and the mysterious healing powers of nature.

A question that remains, however, is how did spa visitors regard the physicians there. Late nineteenth-century diarists and letter-writers remain as reticent about intimate physical matters as in preceding decades, so as in previous chapters, literary sources must be enlisted to offer some tentative answers. The late nineteenth century produced, naturally, its share of humorous or satirical works on the spa experience. In 1860, Heinrich Hoffmann had lampooned the entire practice of spa medicine as

---

[87] Gerhard Rudolph, "100 Jahre wissenschaftliche Balneologie." Keynote Lecture at the 83rd Congress of the Deutsche Gesellschaft für Physikalische Medizin und Rehabilitation, October 13, 1978 in Berlin, reproduced in Gerhard Rudolph, *Zwei Beiträge zur Geschichte der Balneologie* (Kassel: Verlag Hans Meister KG, 1982), 47.

[88] Gerhard Rudolph, "100 Jahre wissenschaftliche Balneologie," 48.

[89] Gerhard Rudolph, "100 Jahre wissenschaftliche Balneologie," 42.

[90] Gerhard Rudolph, "100 Jahre wissenschaftliche Balneologie," 46.

little more than mercenary charlatanism. Had spa medicine made any progress by the end of the century?

Humorous, light entertainment works about spa visits from the late nineteenth century exist, but in each example the character of the physician is nearly absent.[91] This disappearance is significant, suggesting that either doctors and medicine had ceased to be of any relevance at all in spas, or that the figure of the physician had moved from the realm of farce into a more weighty position. An examination of more serious works of literature illuminates the spa experience in a much more meaningful manner, and lend strong support to the latter hypothesis.

Doktor Biebers Versuchung [Doctor Bieber's Temptation], an early novella written by Heinrich Mann in 1898, is set in a private sanatorium in an unspecified spa town.[92] The central figure, Doctor Bieber, the young head doctor at a sanatorium, arrived several years before the narrative begins and quickly took over the leading position from an older, and differently charactered physician, Doctor Westermann. In the words of Herr Sägemüller, a self-described professional neurasthenic who had seen patients at the sanatorium come and go, "Westermann is a fine man, but really far too simple and without deceit. And so there is really nothing fascinating about him. ... Bieber possesses on the other hand a sure feel for the necessary authority. Oh, he has so much more!"[93]

Bieber exuded not simply confidence, but mystery. Sägemüller felt this was in part his art of deception, leading patients, especially women suffering from nervous disorders, to believe in his inexplicable powers, including telekinesis. "With Doctor Bieber one lands inevitably in the realm of the secret, the vague, the half, the inexpressible."[94] Not simply an ordinary physician, Bieber was at the same time a spiritualist and a hypnotist, integrating an element of the occult into his practice. Herein lay the key of Bieber's appeal. Not only was he a healer, but he offered a bridge into a world of transcendental mysticism.

Bieber's power was also essential to the appeal of the sanatorium, which became much more successful after his arrival. He "in his endearing relentlessness resembled a savior and a judge. How monstrously strong

---

[91] See Ewald Altendorf, *Der Badereise* (Berlin: Hesperus Verlag, 1912), or Karl Böttcher, *Karlsbader Schlendertage. Bilder aus dem Saisonleben* (Karlsbad and Nice: Verlag von Hans Feller, 1884).

[92] Heinrich Mann, *Doctor Biebers Versuchung*. in *Gesammelte Werke*, Sigrid Anger, Volker Riedel, eds. (Berlin und Weimar: Aufbau-Verlag, 1978), 16: 453-505.

[93] *Doctor Biebers Versuchung*, 459.

[94] *Doctor Biebers Versuchung*, 460.

was the position of a physician!"[95] This power made the sanatorium into a refuge from the strains of the modern world, fulfilling a role similar to that of a monastery in centuries past. In Sägemüller's words:

> The intellectual person had never stood on a particularly good footing with raw reality, but today we can hardly save ourselves from it, it crowds us inside our houses and outside, too. The electric streetcar that, without my even knowing it, silently glides toward me, meddles in my life as shamelessly as the telephone lines that buzz over my bedroom window at night. Advertising on the corner and the screaming of businessmen and the press, bells everywhere, bicycles and automobiles, I have to endure the rape of my senses by all that, I am helpless against it. Consider also, that the conditions of our material life have grown more and more complicated, but also our intellectual organization has become endlessly more refined. But for the contemporary, much more sensitive intellectual worker there are no longer the places of retreat that earlier, much more coarse learned persons enjoyed. That is why you see me here. The Nerve Clinic is a place of refuge, where I am at last free from the concern of physical existence. As much as possible, I have abdicated my will into the hands of the doctor, and you cannot believe how much good it does a so-called modern man not to need to want anything anymore.[96]

The sanatorium, then, and Doctor Bieber, offered a haven from responsibility, from pressure, from stress. The key element here is surrender of one's will into the authoritative hands of a physician. The character of Bieber, a young physician of a new generation, embodies elements of both the rational and the irrational, of science and of the occult, and therein was the key to his power.

Thomas Mann, Heinrich's younger brother, was also no stranger to spas either in his fictions or his life. Although spas and sanatoria figure in several of his novels, none surpass the depiction in the literary *tour de force*, *The Magic Mountain*. As a literary work *The Magic Mountain* is rich enough to offer endless interpretive possibilities. Science and medicine in the *Magic Mountain*, however, have not often been the subject of analysis, literary or historical, and at times have been dismissed as "a mere property of realistic representation."[97] Mann had clearly done his

---

[95] *Doctor Biebers Versuchung*, 471.
[96] *Doktor Biebers Versuchung*, 479.
[97] Malte Herwig, "Magic Science on the Mountain: Science and Myth in Thomas Mann's *Der Zauberberg*. *Germanic Review* 74, no. 2 (Spring, 1999): 146-156. OCLC FirstSearch HTML version, p 4.

homework, researching medical therapies and procedures in order to arrive at the most realistic representation possible.[98]

First published in 1924, *The Magic Mountain* was conceived and begun following a brief visit to the Swiss resort of Davos in 1912. In a lecture delivered at Princeton University in May 1939, Mann admitted an autobiographical component to the inception of *The Magic Mountain.* Like the protagonist Hans Castorp, Mann did not come to Davos as a patient, but to visit his wife Katia, who was receiving treatment for a lung condition. He recounts being told by a physician that he should remain for half a year for a cure and adds, "if I had followed his advice, I might still be up there."[99] Ten days proved sufficient time for him to shape his experiences of the spa into a compelling representation of the milieu, its patients, and physicians.

Castorp, unlike his creator, did not escape, instead becoming ensnared by the complex net of illness, beauty, and science. This begins when he is introduced to Dr. Krokowski, a physician at the *Berghof* sanatorium. To the doctor's inquiry as to whether he would be staying as a patient, he responded that he was only visiting, and that he was, "thank God, entirely healthy."

> "Truly?" asked Dr. Krokowski, in that he thrust his head forward and askance, as if teasingly, and broadened his smile … "But then you are phenomenon most worth studying! As a matter of fact, I have never seen an entirely healthy person. … And you will not take advantage of any medical treatment here, physical or psychological?"
>
> "No, thank you a thousand times!" said Hans Castorp and nearly took a step backward.
>
> Then Dr. Krokowski's smile broke out again victoriously, and as he shook the young man's hand again, he called out in a loud voice:
>
> "Well, then, sleep well, Mr. Castorp, in the full knowledge of your flawless health! Sleep well, and *auf Wiedersehen!*"[100]

Auf Wiedersehen it was. Castorp comes down with a cold. Those around him, however, obsessed with fever curves, persuade him to see the physician again. This time he sees *Hofrat* [Court Counsellor] Behrens, who determines that the young man is in fact, not merely affected by a minor infection, but rather bears traces of earlier, serious tuberculosis of

[98] Herwig, "Magic Science on the Mountain," p. 4.

[99] Thomas Mann, "Einführung in den Zauberberg für Studenten der Universität Princeton," in Thomas Mann, *Der Zauberberg* (Berlin: Deutsche Buch-Gemeinschaft, 1967), iii.

[100] Thomas Mann, *Der Zauberberg*, 23.

which he had been unaware. In the spa, the *Hofrat* explained to him, latent illness is first aroused, then it can be cured. Dazzled by the show of expertise, Castorp begins to believe. The moment of truth, however, comes during the radiological examination. Ensconced in a dark chamber was the, at the time, high technology equipment mastered by the physician and *Hofrat* Behrens, unleashing the "frightful force"[101] at his disposal. Appropriately impressed, Castorp is ready to see the results. Seeing his cousin's heart on the x-ray film, Castorp filled with awe, with "reflection and shock" sputters out "Yes, yes, I see ... my God, I see!" He saw mortality, and felt in his heart "feelings of being moved and of piety"[102]

Both works by the Mann brothers link physicians with extraordinary, even magical powers that evoke feelings of awe and fear among patients. The physician, as a scientist, has assumed the position of a modern shaman–he holds the keys to arcane knowledge, the secrets of health, and with it, a certain power over life and death.[103] Castorp is initiated into this world in the radiological chamber with *Hofrat* Behrens, the solid medical man, guiding him on his journey. Bieber, although a much more ambiguous character, is even more shrouded in mystery. And, of course, to the uninitiated patient, mystery is the source of the doctor's power.

Regarded allegorically, the magic of the *Berghof*, and the power of Doctor Bieber's spell lay not in the occult, nor in the enchantment of the mountains, but in the power of medical knowledge. How, though, is this different from Romantic spa physicians claiming to harness the powers of nature? In the late nineteenth century, most of mainstream science had accepted the limits of knowledge, rejecting comprehensive systems and ultimate answers in favor of specialization in particular fields of knowledge and concrete questions. Serious science limited itself in its questions. Balneologists, like other physicians, tried to restrict their field in this manner in order to give it greater gravity as a field and to free it from traces of natural philosophy and any hint of mysticism.

So why, then, does magic figure so prominently in these two works? Herein lies the paradox. Although science could not answer all questions, and skepticism about the powers of science grew especially after 1900, the general acceptance of the scientific world-view prevalent in the late nineteenth century bolstered the physician's authority. For middle-class laymen, including engineers, lawyers, businessmen and philologists, the

[101] Thomas Mann, *Der Zauberberg*, 226.
[102] Thomas Mann, *Der Zauberberg*, 229.
[103] For a discussion of the scientist as a modern shaman, see Malte Herwig, "Magic Science on the Mountain."

scientific approach was largely an accepted norm.[104] This is especially clear in German. An attorney specialized in the science of laws [*Rechtswissenschaft*], a businessman followed and used the science of economics [*Wirtschaftswissenschaft*], and each recognized the specialization of his field. So, too, then, a physician was recognized as the specialist in the area of health, the science of medicine. Medicine, however, is associated with existential questions, ultimately of human nature and of mortality, questions that defy complete explanation. Paradoxically, then, the physician, as the master of medical science, was also the keeper of arcane knowledge, and hence, metaphorically speaking, possessed a nearly supernatural power as well.

In an era when technological advancement and social upheaval, in which life's certainties suddenly seemed far less certain –the Age of Anxiety –surrendering oneself to the direction of a physician, especially in a remote and peaceful spa, could offer relief from a stress-filled existence . The spa physician, to a greater extent than his clinical counterparts, could claim explicitly or implicitly to bridge science and the wonder of nature. As a serious scientist and researcher, an image consciously cultivated by balneologists, he earned the respect of rational, thinking people. Simultaneously, however, his exclusive understanding of that science, his ability to use water and air to heal, or at least the belief that he could, made him something mysterious and awesome, not merely a man of science, but a magician.

But therein lay the crux of the issue. Spa physicians, wielding the elemental forces of nature, could be seen as magicians. This made them an interesting literary subject, a figure to be held in awe. At the same time, however, balneology, tainted by this hint of "magic" remained on the fringe of academic medicine. To be sure, specialists had organized into professional associations, and balneology was included in university medical school curricula, but wholehearted acceptance remained, and remains today, elusive. The partial successes of the late nineteenth century did not continue. In the twentieth century, the efficacy of balneological therapy in treating serious disease was not convincingly established. While other disciplines made real therapeutic advances, balneology did not, and perhaps could not, keep pace. By the 1990s, a German medical student

---

[104] For a discussion of the role of science in late nineteenth century German society, see Thomas Nipperdey, *Deutsche Geschichte, 1866-1918*, (Munich: C.H. Beck, 1998), 1: 602-691.

might be taunted with the obviously demeaning prospect of not finding a position in a hospital and becoming “only a spa physician.”[105]

[105] Author’s own conversations with medical students and staff physicians in the Department of Radiology at the University of Tübingen, 1992.

CHAPTER SIX

CONCLUSIONS

The nineteenth century was a golden age for health spas. By the turn of the twentieth century, they enjoyed an unprecedented popularity, evidenced by their ever-rising visitor statistics. The goals stated by spa administrations such as the Cure Committee of Baden-Baden at the outset of the century, making over the town into a popular and respected resort and a revenue-producing enterprise, had been achieved in striking measure. The same could be said for many other spas of international stature, such as Wiesbaden and Bad Ems, but also of smaller resorts with a more local clientele, such as Bad Kissingen and Wildbad. Spas became a growth industry in nineteenth-century Germany, proliferating widely across forested hillside landscapes, and sought out by an ever larger number of patrons for their presumed regenerative powers and pleasures. Emerging from the aristocratic, court-oriented gathering places of the eighteenth century, spas were by 1914 essentially commercial enterprises selling health and relaxation to a largely, although certainly not entirely, middle-class public. As this study has endeavored to show, the grand spas were successful, not only because they offered a stylish destination for a weary public in search of recreation, but because they promised healing and convalescence to patrons with a multitude of illnesses, physical and psychological.

Success was in part the result of the modern promotional techniques of the spa administrations. These tended to emphasize the medical value of the spas and their waters together with the restorative quality of the natural environment, testififying both to the influential position of spa physicians in determining the form such promotion would take, and also answering to the desires of the curing public. Visitor statistics throughout the century show a clear upward trend for the grand spas. With the exception of times of social crisis, such as 1848/49, the wars of the 1860s and 1870/71, and the financial crash of 1873, the number of guests hosted in the elegant resort towns consistently grew if not year for year, at least decade by decade.

Numbers of visitors reveal little, however, about what attracted them, and what they did upon arrival. No doubt, many came solely for leisure and social hobnobbing. Such, after all, was the reputation of the spa, especially at mid-century, as a place where the wealthy came to be pampered, to connect for social advancement, business purposes, or romantic adventures. What, then, of the spas' own assertions, as advanced most vociferously by spa physicians, that they were places of refuge from a hectic world in which serious medicine was practiced?

This study bears out the essential truth of this claim. The pattern of infrastructure expansion, and the resources lavished upon this activity, offers compelling evidence that the spas were indeed perceived as serious medical establishments. Spa administrations raised impressive new edifices at regular intervals over the course of the entire century. Baden-Baden, the spa examined in the greatest detail here, expanded its Conversation House in 1808, constructed a new one in 1823, a new steam bath and a new Pump Room (*Trinkhalle*) in 1816 and 1822 respectively; both were replaced again around 1850, a monumental steam bath was erected in 1873 and a second such bath for women was added in 1892. Nor was Baden-Baden unique in this respect. Wiesbaden and Ems, two other successful spas, followed a similar construction schedule.

Analysis of the decision-making process reveals that each modernization was undertaken by the spa administration to meet the needs of the curing public, as it perceived them, in order to make the spa more attractive for potential visitors. The calculations of the bureaucrats were essentially correct: the new fixtures and structures filled up during the season, and at a fairly regular interval of approximately thirty years, patron demand outstripped their capacities, requiring something bigger and better in their place. Had visitors not been interested in much more than elegant soirées and high-stakes casino gaming, in social positioning, courtship liaisons, and discreet encounters, such costly investment in infrastructure would have made no sense. With impressive consistency, the spa administration, itself a collection of competing interests and competencies, correctly interpreted the nature of consumer-patron demand over the short and long term.

One could, of course, adopt a supply-side perspective on the question and contend that a new Pump Room or bathhouse created demand for itself that had not existed previously. Perhaps, the novelty of the amenity explains the growing number of visitors. Such a hypothesis, however, runs counter to archival evidence, which shows in each case that the spa administration acted in response to desires expressed by visitors and by physicians wishing to expand their practice (and expecting to do so on the basis of physical improvements). Especially after steamships and railroads gave travelers a new ease of mobility, in the highly competitive and elastic spa market, patrons could easily, and did actually, take their business to another spa offering services which they felt better suited their needs. Supply, in this case, responded to demand, and not vice versa.

Unique to the spa as a medical institution, from its early modern beginnings, was the complimentary amalgamation of healing and leisure in one environment, with both being an integral part of the experience. Throughout the century, spa patrons sought a balance between amusement and the spa's ostensible *raison d'etre*, curing. In order to be appealing to the widest possible range of clients, spas had to offer something for everyone with the means at their disposal to take a curative, to go on a *Badereise*. For some, this meant luxury, for others, a chance to gamble, for others still, a cure. Baden-Baden and Wiesbaden enjoyed such popularity and renown as they were perhaps the most successful, with state sponsorship and lavish funding available from casino proceeds, in providing a full range of services in the most up-to date and urbane environs.

Nevertheless, these refined refuges earned dubious reputations in the eyes of the moralistically-inclined because of their "seductive iniquity." The most objectionable feature of course was the casino. Shocking tales of elderly ladies squandering their children's inheritance at the roulette wheel or of young innocents losing first their money, then their virtue at the green tables, fired the indignation of authors in the pages of the middle-class *Morgenblatt*. Driven, perhaps, by such sensational stories, the moral opprobrium, especially among the core market of the middle classes, grew to a point that steps had to be taken. That agitation to prohibit gaming in spas intensified as middle-class visitors became preponderant was a fact that spa administrations could not ignore. Elegance and social spectacle the *bourgeois* could countenance, even relish, but the aristocratic pastime of high-stakes gambling, seen by many as morally degenerate, could not be tolerated in what was becoming in increasing measure a middle-class institution.

The first major attempt to cure German spas of the infirmity of casino gaming came from the Frankfurt Parliament in 1849, but the ban was swept aside along with the Parliament itself. Prohibition came with German unification, which ushered in a new era in the world of German spas as well. The period after the last casino was shut down in 1872 was a test of the spas' real attractive power and endurance. Many shared the Russian novelist Turgenev's gloomy vision of its inevitable demise. Yet not all were so morose. In particular spa physicians saw a golden opportunity. Baden-Baden and Wiesbaden, representative of the cosmopolitan German spas, wagered their future on a shift in focus back to their waters. Impressive ultra-modern bathhouses, it was hoped, would attract the public and keep them coming back season after season. Once the economy recovered from the economic doldrums of the 1870s and Germans again had more disposable income, the spas quickly regained and then surpassed their former popularity, even though French guests, an important part of the pre-war curing public, boycotted the spas of their German conquerors. The waters and the impressive bathhouses, it seems, were more than enough to make patrons forget the roulette wheel.

Balneologists had always claimed that curing was paramount in the spa. With the casino gone, their claims could be tested and upheld. By the early 1870s, there could no longer be any doubt that the waters were the major draw for visitors. The existence of gambling may have obscured what had always been the case, however. Teplitz and Karlsbad in the Austrian Empire had survived and even prospered without the lure of gaming, even though they had been outstripped in popularity by spas that allowed it, such as Baden-Baden and Wiesbaden. But demand for water cures had noticeably intensified as early as the 1840s, as suggested by the rapid proliferation of new spas, and Priessnitz-inspired water institutes. Gambling was simply not the essential factor in explaining which spas thrived and which did not. The fundamental forces determining a particular spa's success or failure were far less beholden to chance than that: ample state sponsorship, assertive promotional efforts, especially among physicians, and broad advertising campaigns alerting the public to all the important benefits and pleasures to be had from a *Badereise.*

Promotion in this competitive market was geared toward gaining the greatest market share possible, and consequently, the strategies used reflected the priorities and desires of the times. Themes that were constantly emphasized throughout the century were the relaxing power of the natural environment. Claim as they may that their mineral springs offered unique healing properties, spa promoters had to recognize that these assertions were virtually nullified by the similar declarations of a host of rivals. As a result, the unique ambiance and pleasures of a given locale was recruited in the advertising effort. This was by no means a contradiction or a sign that physicians in fact believed that all mineral waters were the same; rather, in order to allow patients to benefit from their wondrous waters (and physicians' private practices), they had to be drawn to the spa by whatever means possible. Consequently, equally consistent, and often more prominent in the promotional literature was a focus on the amusements to be found in a given spa. These were tailored to prevailing trends, e.g. caves and ruins during the Romantic period, as well as the much-touted spa freedom, supplanted later by a greater appeal to the possibilities of social networking of various kinds. The essence of these promotional efforts did not change much over the century, but should be viewed more as variations on a theme: amusement and distraction to facilitate healing.

What did change significantly, however, was the manner in which the medical aspect of the spa was advertised. This reflected changes in medical thought rather than the direct economic interest of the promoters. Medical advertising until the 1850s was dominated by Romantic natural philosophy, emphasizing the mysterious and unfathomable healing powers of the waters, and laying claim to vast efficaciousness. After 1850, however, influenced by developments toward a more scientific-experimental medicine and greater skepticism among a more educated public, a gradual but clear shift to specialist spas became evident. By 1870 and thereafter, no spa dared tout its waters or its healers as being able to cure any condition imaginable, but now focused on a few –still an impressively large few, it is true –ailments for which its springs were best suited.

This development in advertising mirrored the internal shift within spa medicine itself. Where in 1830 spa physicians saw themselves as generalists with a particular skill in exploiting the mysterious life-force contained in the waters, by 1880 they were struggling for respect as members of an advanced medical specialty: balneology. The replacement of the term "spa doctor" (*Badearzt*) with "balneologist" (*Balneologe*) also corresponded, tellingly enough, to a change in tone toward patients. One could expect that a more specialized physician, in essence a more modern professional, would adopt a more authoritarian tone in addressing patients.

Early spa physicians urged readers of their guides to always consult a physician, threatening them with examples of the horrid consequences of not seeking and scrupulously following expert medical advice, and admonishing them to never attempt a self-cure under any circumstances. In a seeming contradiction of their own advice, they then proceeded to equip readers with the knowledge necessary to do precisely this. The shift became apparent after 1850, when first warnings appeared about consulting non-specialists, i.e., non-balneologists, and then finally, after 1880, virtually all such warnings disappeared from the literature and few details about the therapies themselves were divulged. Prevalent instead were advertisements inviting potential patients to speak to their regular physicians.

In this sense, and in many others, spa physicians were emulating the professional development toward specialization and adopting the same strategies to establish their authority as those pursued by mainstream physicians. It would appear, then, that spa doctors had been vindicated. By 1880, their long-time dream of making curing the center of the spa experience and themselves the sole determinants of treatment had been largely fulfilled. The spa towns were flourishing. They no longer needed to admonish patients not to treat themselves, but could evidently rest fairly assured that they were at long last regarded as *the* experts in their field, the keepers of specialist knowledge. Yet the complete picture was not so rosy or unambiguous.

Spa physicians followed the general pattern of other physicians, defining themselves as a specialist field represented by professional organizations that advocated their causes. In this, however, they lagged behind other fields of medicine, always having to struggle against the suspicions that surrounded their specialty and which stood in the way of the respect and admiration they were sure they deserved. They never fully succeeded, but remained, more or less, marginal to mainstream medicine, unable fully to convince their colleagues of the scientific gravity of their field.

In this sense, balneologists inhabited a grey zone between their colleagues in other branches of medicine and the growing number of alternative practitioners such as homeopaths, naturopaths, and lay healers, who questioned the bases of modern laboratory medicine. By the 1880s, balneologists in large part no longer doubted the fundamentals of allopathic medicine, but embraced them, asserting that the mineral waters at their disposal were a useful and effective therapy. By 1914, they could reflect on some considerable success in penetrating, or remaining in the medical establishment as represented in university teaching curricula. Many balneologists were at the same time specialists in diverse fields such as physiology, pharmacology, or surgery. Yet even in their own scientific deliberations, they never could entirely dispense with the echoes of Romantic natural philosophy. The *Brunnengeist* or life-force of Romantic medicine might be transmuted into mineral compounds or later, radioactivity, yet still they could not fully erase the lingering suspicions about their credentials.

As a professional group, recipients of the same university training as other physicians, struggling for recognition as credible scientists while keeping alternative practitioners, lay healers and outright quacks at bay, balneologists represented a group of insider-outsiders. Having earned university degrees in medicine, they were decidedly not laymen, like Priessnitz or Kneipp. They were unrelenting in their efforts to drive out unlicensed competitors who might undermine their reputation. These efforts were only partially successful, because they themselves could never completely shed the taint of their origins in natural philosophy. The undiscriminating public continued to associate them with lay healers. When balneologists periodically attempted to co-opt their competitors by adopting and adapting their methods, they only added to the popular confusion.

Their failure to win an equal place in the first ranks of the medical practice says much about the development of medicine and medical authority in Germany. Balneologists were in fact physicians, and as late nineteenth-century university teaching programs testify, the field was regarded as a legitimate discipline of academic medicine, not as an alternative one outside of the pale of academic medicine. By virtue of their insider-outsider status, one may argue that balneologists' actions were highly indicative of trends and attitudes within medicine as a whole. As those with partial membership, and a longing to belong fully to the established group of academic physicians, they spared no effort to do what was necessary to gain full insider status within the establishment medical world.

Their strategies are revealing. Authority issued from specialization. To this end, balneologists, like the colleagues in other fields, formed a successful professional association in 1889, the autonomous *Balneologische Gesellschaft*. They readily made use of state power to bolster their authority and position, as exemplified by the police harassment of presumed quacks, and by the consistent police verification of medical credentials in Baden-Baden. In this practice, they were better situated than their mainstream colleagues because their spa practices often contributed directly to the revenues of the state. After mid-century, spa physicians promoted themselves as specialists in a scientific discipline of the post-Virchow sense. The development of spa physicians into balneologists closely paralleled, with some delay, that of other academically trained physicians.[1]

---

[1] Studies in the professionalization of medicine have consistently overlooked balneologists as a branch of the profession, either excluding them entirely, or subsuming them into a larger group of physicians. The reason for this may lie in the contemporary ahistorical perception of balneology as pseudoscience and not serious medicine. See for example Claudia Huerkamp, *Der Aufstieg der Ärzte 19. Jahrhundert* (Göttingen, Vanderhoeck & Ruprecht, 1985), or from the patient-centered viewpoint, Jens Lachmund, Gunnar Stollberg, *Patientenwelten: Krankheit und Medizin vom späten 18. bis zum frühen 20. Jahrhundert im Spiegel von Autobiographien* (Opladen: Leske & Budrich, 1995).

Yet in one critical area of the professionalization of medicine in Germany, the role of public health insurance in the establishment of professional authority, balneologists working in spas such as Baden-Baden diverged radically from their counterparts. A major element of the most common professionalization thesis is that German physicians at last were able to attain professional autonomy, not through professional organizations or the efficacy of their therapies, which remained limited until the twentieth century, but through the financial security that resulted from a steady stream of patients. The regulations of German health insurance legislation, not their own efforts, were what made this possible. As Claudia Huerkamp most notably argues, by liberating physicians from the need to pander to wealthy patrons, as had been the case for centuries, compulsory health insurance ensured physicians a steady income, which in turn enabled them to assert their authority.

This theory, however, exhibits serious shortcomings when applied to balneologists. Consistent with the policy of social segregation practiced at least since the beginning of the nineteenth century, insurance patients in the grand spas were shunted off into public facilities such as the *Landesbad* in Baden-Baden, and denied full access to the amenities of the town. Even with such a public clinic, insurance patients made up only a small portion of the spa's guests, and could hardly guarantee the balneologist a respectable income. The vast majority of medical practice in Baden-Baden, as illustrated by the fee structure of private sanatoria, was closed to the insurance patient, and remained the domain of private practitioners and private patients who paid cash for their services.

Yet even in this island of private, fee-based practice, medical authority blossomed and expanded, and this was not simply a result of the fact that physicians constituted a substantial part of the spa administration. Indirect evidence, such as the nature of medical promotional efforts in which balneologists seemed confident that patients would consult a specialist, is supported by the growth of private sanatoria, in which patients voluntarily submitted to the authority of a physician. Literature from the period, while not as reliable as the direct testimony such as letters or diaries, rounds out the image: the spa physician, without the support of insurance funds, was able not only to attract patients, but to gain their acceptance of his authority as an expert in medical knowledge.

What should be clear from the preceding chapters is that balneologists did not regard themselves as alternative medicine in the vein of homeopaths or osteopaths. Their training, and their professional associations and assertions, consistently emphasized that they were part of mainstream, academic medicine, not an alternative to it. How patients perceived them is more difficult to ascertain, and would be worthy of even more detailed investigation than has been possible here. The fact remains, however, that balneologists behaved as, portrayed themselves as, and honestly believed themselves to be full-fledged members of the medical establishment. As such, they were able to establish successful practices and private sanatoria in spa towns, which drew tens of thousands of paying visitors annually.

Medicine, by the late nineteenth century, was a large component of the appeal of spas, although not the only one. It is beyond doubt that fashion, luxury, and scenery had considerable power to attract guests to the spa. This was true in 1805, and was still the case a century later. Yet the choice of location for these leisure settings, a salubrious environment that offered mineral springs, is significant, and indicates an enduring link between health and leisure. Why, however, did so many spa patrons seek to do so under the direction of a physician? As with any question of mentality, the answers are complex and incomplete, yet this study suggests several possibilities. In increasing measure, through agitation, education, and popularization of science, health and preventative hygiene grew to be linked not only with bourgeois respectability, but with nationalism and patriotism. The *Friedrichsbad* in Baden-Baden played on this theme, linking state-of-the art curing and national grandeur in one edifice. To care for one's health, to be hygienically clean in body and mind, was a positive act, not simply for one's self, but more importantly, for the nation as a whole. Doctors may have encouraged this attitude, but nationalism was a much more potent incentive to which they could only contribute. "Promoting the health of the nation," no doubt, contributed in turn to their own authority.

Another factor lay in the hectic nature of industrial civilization. By the end of the century, nervous afflictions of all kinds, once only the privilege of the affluent, seemed to have reached epidemic proportions. The widespread diagnosis of neurasthenia proved a boon for the spa. Anxiety, tension, nervousness were exactly the kind of intangible symptoms that spa treatment had always inclined to. Now, an individual could surrender his or her will to an expert physician, in order to do something constructive and beneficial in a refuge away from all the frightening tensions of the age. As one's personal responsibilities grew, so too did the need to escape them, to become passive, in the literal meaning of the word "patient." "Not to need to want anything," in the words of one of Heinrich Mann's characters, even or especially the need to make decisions, must have been a powerful lure. Of course, one could not simply abandon responsibility or go off to some distant island. Escape could only be temporary and it required guidance; otherwise, to the rest of the world and to oneself it might look too much like an impermissible self-indulgence. The physician, commanding the powers of new and impressive science, in a realm both remote *and* well-regulated, stood ready to use his expertise to effect a cure. To some, he might well appear to be a beneficent magician.

At least as important as patient need was the growing adulation for medicine as a natural science, which contributed significantly to the increase in physicians' authority. Specialization in medicine, as this study has suggested, was linked with medicalization and the growth of medical authority. Throughout the nineteenth century, physicians asserted that their expertise entitled them to respect and admiration, and to this pattern spa physicians were no exception. It was only with the supplanting of the generalist by the specialist in the final decades of the century that medical doctors acquired their longed-for status and authority. This was not simply a question of power and financial independence acquired through practices filled with insurance patients, but perhaps more significantly though a deep change in mentality.[2] Spa patients, financing their own cures, willingly chose to submit to a physician.

Medicalization, as this history of the German spa shows, must be regarded as an interactive process. The interpretation that the position of "patient," being both subject of and to the medical gaze, was imposed by physicians acting in close conjunction with the state through the process of professionalization provides only a partial explanation. Doctors did in fact wish to impose their wills, to give orders and to be obeyed as unquestioningly as military commanders. Yet medical doctors craved this recognition of their authority already in 1805. Spa doctors had had intimate relations with various German states for nearly a century without having achieved their heart's desire. The ability to command patient respect and obedience, it seems reasonable to surmise, must have resulted from changes in patients' mindset as well. Such changes of attitude cannot be dictated by professionals or by the state. They have complicated histories. For middle-class spa patients, the doctor came by the turn of the twentieth century to be a trusted expert in science, to whose authority one's will could be temporarily surrendered. The reward for those who could afford it was a true vacation from the difficult nineteenth century.

---

[2] Hans-Ulrich Wehler, *Deutsche Gesellschaftsgeschichte, Band 3: Von der "Deutschen Doppelrevolution" bis zum Beginn des Ersten Weltkrieges, 1849-1914* (Munich: C.H. Beck, 1995, p. 738.

CHAPTER SEVEN

EPILOGUE

By 1914, at the end of the long nineteenth century, German health spas and spa physicians could look back over the previous century with a considerable and justified sense of satisfaction. Their greatest fears in that fateful summer were likely questions of how to maintain their success. The Great War, however, brought the long nineteenth century to a close, and the peace of 1919 plunged them into a new reality they could not have anticipated.

Sir Edward Grey's oft-quoted observation that the lamps went out in Europe in August 1914 was certainly true for the spas. War did not destroy them–they continue until the present day–but something of the cosmopolitan atmosphere was indeed lost, no longer sustainable in a Europe awash in chauvinism. Resorts such as Baden-Baden were mobilized as military hospitals for the convalescence of wounded, gassed, and shell-shocked troops.

The convalescence of the spas themselves during the 1920s required radical adjustments to a new reality. Gone was the mystique of elegance and the world of aristocratic trappings; neither seemed appropriate in the aftermath of so much death and suffering. The fledgling Republic provided no fitting environment for a return to past glories. In 1933, the Nazis, badly in need of revenue, reinstated what had been lost in 1872: Baden-Baden was allowed to re-open its casino as the only one in Germany. Visitor statistics soared, and for a time it may have seemed that the fine days of the past had returned. A promotional film from the mid-1930s certainly tried to present this image. Yet the film, despite the filmmakers best efforts, could not hide the lackluster, down-at-the-heels establishment. [1] Renovated again in 1934, the Conversation House may have been filled with dancers as over 100,000 visitors came annually to

[1] StA BB, uncatalogued promotional film for Baden-Baden, ca. 1935.

the spa,[2] but the erstwhile brilliance, lively expectations, and elegance had been irrevocably lost with the end of the era.

It was not that the Nazis took any particular interest in spas *per se*. Baden-Baden, with over fifteen percent of its guests once again coming from abroad, was meant to function largely as an international showcase for the new regime. Consequently, the town was, for a time at least, spared the Nazi policies that might have offended or shocked foreign guests. The authorities allowed Baden-Baden to remain open to Jewish guests until as late as January 1937, when after four years of constant growth and a doubling of the number of visitors, *Gauleiter* Robert Wagner followed the example of other spas, and ordered the exclusion of all Jews from the spa's amenities.[3] This was not a sudden development, nor was it a Nazi invention. The Third Reich merely completed a process of excluding Jews from public accommodations, hotels, seaside resorts, and spas that was already decades old by 1937.

Systematic expressions of antisemitism in German spas have been traced back to the late nineteenth century, beginning on a small scale with individual hotels and restaurants which advertised themselves as "*judenfrei,*" then growing in scope, especially after 1918, as entire resorts made it clear that Jews were not welcome. Germany was not the only country in which such exclusion was evident: many vacation spots in the United States had a clear policy of being closed to Jewish guests. One historian has estimated that a much higher percentage of spas in the United States excluded Jews than in Germany prior to 1933. Germany, however, was unique, not only for the obvious fact that it alone produced the Nazis and ultimately the Holocaust, but in the radical ideological quality of the policies.[4]

Prior to the advent of the Nazis, however, the grand spas, the subject for this study, were largely free from institutionalized antisemitism, unlike many smaller spas and seaside resorts. A few hotels in the largely southern German spas advertised their "Christian character," indirectly indicating that Jews were not welcome, but these represented isolated exceptions to a generally more cosmopolitan atmosphere.[5] Spa policies with regard to

---

[2] Rolf-Gustav Haebler, *Geschichte der Stadt und des Kurortes Baden-Baden*, Second Edition (Baden-Baden: Verlag Dr. Willy Schmidt, 1969), 2: 187.

[3] Frank Bajohr, "*Unser Hotel ist judenfrei." Bäder-Antisemitismus im 19. und 20. Jahrhundert*. (Frankfurt am Main: Fischer Taschenbuchverlag), 2003, 127-128.

[4] For a full and richly documented study of this aspect of the history of spas, see Bajohr, *"Unser Hotel ist judenfrei."*

[5] Bajohr, *"Unser Hotel ist judenfrei,"* 20. In addition to the advertising of individual establishments, a small number of guidebooks were published in order to lead

Jewish (and at times also Catholic) guests varied greatly, but there was little systematic discrimination, and by no account a general policy of exclusion.[6] This stood in stark contrast to many Northern German seaside resorts and several smaller Bavarian spas, where overt antisemitism moved from lampooning of Jewish guests to outright prohibition, most notably in Zinnowitz and Heiligenhafen, which had "pioneered" the antisemitic exclusion of Jews as early as the 1880s, with a host of other Baltic and Thuringian resorts following suit by the outbreak of World War One.[7] In contrast, the island resorts of Norderney, along with classic spas such as Baden-Baden and Wiesbaden, had a tradition reaching back at least to the 1850s of Kosher Jewish hotels, synagogues, and a generally open and tolerant atmosphere.[8]

The research conducted for this study found only a few references to overt antisemitic behavior.[9] On the other hand, archival records do suggest an attitude of openness and tolerance, and even hostility toward antisemitic attitudes among the spa administrators. As early as 1805, in the era before Jewish emancipation, there were at least two hotels in Baden-Baden open to Jews, which hosted over seven percent of all visitors that year.[10] Thereafter, the category of "Jewish inn" disappears from the records, as do all references to whether visitors were Jewish or gentile; only country of origin continued as a category. A century later, by which time a movement to exclude Jews from spas and seaside resorts was underway, Baden-Baden clearly was not "Jew-free." In 1906, the spa town advertised two inns which offered a Kosher kitchen,[11] a fact which was but

---

antisemitically-minded travellers to the "right" establishments. See *Reise-Handbuch für die christliche Familie. Ein Wegweiser durch Hospize, Erholungshäuser, Pensionen, Hotels, Sanatorien, Sommerfrischen, Bäder, Kurorte, nebst praktischen Auskünften für die Reise*, Seventeenth Edition (Berlin: Vaterländische Verlags- und Kunstanstalt, 1912). The classic spas do not figure prominently in this guidebook, as opposed to the resorts where antisemitism was prevalent.

6 Sommer, *Zur Kur nach Ems*, 485 ff.

7 Bajohr, *"Unser Hotel ist judenfrei,"* 19.

8 Bajohr, *"Unser Hotel ist judenfrei,"* 89.

9 See the discussion of the case of the investigation of Dr. Senff in Chapter Five.

10 GLA Ka 195/294, Report of the Spa Commission on the number of visitors, listed by hotel, in the 1805 season, "Gubrauchung der Badkur in Baden sich eingefundenen Fremden," October 7, 1805, in "Bestellung der Badekomission und deren Wirksamkeit zur Emporbringung des Bades. 1805-1808,"

11 StA BB 26-29-173, Advertising flyer for Baden-Baden, "1911 Hotels, Logierhäuser, Pensionen, Sanatorien, und Kur-Anstalten in Baden-Baden (Schwarzwald)," issued by the City Tourism Office, in "Verkehrswesen: Prospekt von Baden-Baden, 1906."

one element of its reputation, which lasted into the 1930s, as one of the so-called "*Judenbäder*."[12] Baden-Baden remained a refuge for Jews until 1937, even as the other grand spas ceased to accept them. Aside from its historic tolerance, Baden-Baden was the sole exception for the reasons mentioned above. The fewer international guests a given spa hosted, the sooner Jews were excluded.

In light of these overt manifestations of antisemitism in many resorts, and the influential position of physicians in shaping policies, the issue of the degree and nature of support for the Nazis to be found among spa physicians is significant. The medical community as a whole was over-represented in the Nazi Movement and, along with lawyers, played a vital role in defining the Third Reich's agenda of "racial hygiene" and implementing the so-called Final Solution of the Jewish Question.[13] Physicians and medical students who joined the party prior to 1933 were frequently, although not always, antisemites, members of the *Freikorps*,

---

[12] Bajohr, *"Unser Hotel ist judenfrei,"* 94.

[13] Michael H. Kater, "Hitler's Early Doctors: Nazi Physicians in Predepression Germany," *Journal of Modern History* 59, no. 1 (March 1987), 29. The scholarly literature on the link between Nazi physicians and genocide is extensive. See Alexander Mitscherlich, Fred Mielke, *Doctors of Infamy; the Story of the Nazi Medical Crimes* (New York: Henry Schuman, 1949); Benno Müller-Hill, *Murderous Science: Elimination by Scientific Selection of Jews, Gypsies, and Others, Germany 1933-1945* (Oxford: Oxford University Press, 1988); Stefan Kühl, *The Nazi Connection: Eugenics, American Racism, and German National Socialism* (New York: Oxford University Press, 1994); Michael Burleigh, *Ethics and Extermination: Reflections on Nazi Genocide* (New York: Cambridge University Press, 1997); Robert Jay Lifton, *The Nazi Doctors: Medical Killing and the Psychology of Genocide* (London: Macmillan, 1986); Paul Weindling, *Health, Race, and German Politics between National Unification and Nazism, 1870-1945* (Cambridge, New York: Cambridge University Press, 1989); Geoffrey Cocks, *Treating Mind and Body: Essays in the History of Science, Professions, and Society under Extreme Conditions* (New Brunswick, NJ: Transaction Publishers, 1998); Robert Proctor, *Racial Hygiene: Medicine under the Nazis* (Cambridge, MA: Harvard University Press, 1988); Francis R. Nicosia, Jonathan Huener, eds., *Medicine and Medical Ethics in Nazi Germany: Origins, Practices, Legacies* (New York: Berghahn Books, 2002); Hans-Walter Schmuhl, *Rassenhygiene, Nationalsozialismus, Euthanasie: von der Verhütung zur Vernichtung "lebensunwerten Lebens," 1890-1945* (Göttingen: Vanderhoeck & Ruprecht, 1987); Henry Friedlander, *The Origins of Nazi Genocide: From Euthanasia to the Final Solution* (Chapel Hill: University of North Carolina Press, 1995); Michael H. Kater, *Doctors under Hitler* (Chapel Hill: University of North Carolina Press, 1989); Aly Götz, Peter Chroust, Christian Pross, *Cleansing the Fatherland: Nazi Medicine and Racial Hygiene* (Baltimore: Johns Hopkins University Press, 1994).

and other radical rightist organizations.[14] Spa physicians, too, were drawn into the Nazi orbit, and some were vocal supporters of Hitler. One such individual, the *Medizinalrat* Emil Vollmer, nearing retirement from his long career as a balneologist practicing in Bad-Kreuznach in 1935, concluded his memoirs with an evidently enthusiastic physician's view of the Nazi future:

> [I]n our era, the faith in a German future is coming again to light… given to us by the miracle of the German leadership of Adolf Hitler, if we only tread the path that he has shown to all Germans with his strong will and clear-sighted optimism. … There is now in the new era of the Third Reich a concern for the health of the nation has become the *völkisch* life force, spreading in all directions, that cares for the healthy growth and unencumbered further development of headstrong Germans. … May an unencumbered development of peace enable Adolf Hitler's new Reich to complete all its plans for the healing of the nation!
>
> Heil Hitler![15]

Such an example, however, is anecdotal and must be taken with a degree of caution. It may or may not have been part of a larger pattern. The relative lack of antisemitism in the spas examined for this study limits the extent to which its findings are useful in reaching any certainty about how prevalent antisemitism was among spa doctors. But, of course, there were reasons, other than antisemitism, prompting spa doctors to support National Socialism and little evidence to suggest that they resisted it in any significant number. Naturally, an economic argument can be brought to bear. Dating back to at least the 1880s, there was a notable hostility toward Jewish physicians on the part of their gentile counterparts. Although efforts to exclude Jewish doctors from medical societies failed, they still faced considerable animosity and discrimination in the Kaiserreich and the Weimar Republic, which grew as physicians' anxiety over heightened competition increased. The elimination of Jewish competition in the medical field, in the context of the "over-production" of doctors in the 1920s, might well have appealed to non-Jewish practitioners, whether they were sincere racists or simply opportunists.[16]

---

[14] Kater, "Hitler's Early Doctors," 30.

[15] Emil Vollmer, *Meine Erinnerungen* (Bad Kreuznach: Harrach, 1935), 74-75.

[16] Michael H. Kater, "Professionalization and Socialization of Physicians in Wilhelmine and Weimar Germany," *Journal of Contemporary History,* 20, no. 4 (October, 1985), 689-90. After 1871, medicine was the most popular course of studies for Jewish university students, and after 1900, second only to law. Overall,

Yet another factor that moved spa physicians to support Nazism was fear of losing their professional autonomy. The specter of collectivism in social insurance, which in the late Weimar period doctors feared would turn them into pauperized salaried employees, combined with a perceived loss of lucrative practices to heighten their status anxiety. Medical students and young practitioners were alarmed over what they saw as shrinking professional opportunities. Despite the Republic's confirmation of doctors' status as an independent, *not* salaried, profession (*freiberuflicher Status*) in 1931, many remained nervous. The Nazis spoke to these worries, promising professional autonomy in a reformed economy based on "moral footings," one that would properly prize the individuality and exclusivity of medical work. With such rhetoric, the *Nationalsozialistischer Deutscher Ärztebund* (National Socialist Association of German Physicians) apparently convinced the majority of physicians.[17]

This study suggests that catering to the spa doctors' sense of autonomy may have been the most effective argument the Nazis could have made. As the record shows, the physicians examined in this work had always craved authority and autonomy, to be respected as experts whose instructions were to be followed and whose abilities trusted unquestioningly. By the end of the nineteenth century, they were to an extent able to acquire these attributes, while remaining largely independent of the state health insurance system. A promise to defend their cherished independence against democratic and socialist interference, and the suggestion that it might be even further fortified by a regime sympathetic to authority, were exactly what most in the profession longed to hear.

Of course, this argument cannot be taken as even approaching a comprehensive account of the phenomenon of Nazi doctors. Aside from implications about a desire for unrestrained authority taken to a macabre extreme, it does nothing to explain the pseudo-scientific experiments in Auschwitz and other concentration camps. Given the complexity of the issue, a wide range of scholarship must be considered. The eugenics and

---

it has been estimated that in 1871, Jews constituted just over one percent of the general population, but ten percent of medical students and five percent of doctors. Jewish physicians were concentrated in major urban centers such as Berlin and Hamburg, where by the turn of the century, they may have accounted for up to one-third of practicing physicians.

[17] Peter Thomsen, *Ärzte auf dem Weg ins "Dritte Reich:" Studien zur Arbeitsmarktsituation, zum Selbstverständnis und zur Standespolitik der Ärzteschaft gegenüber der Sozialversicherung während der Weimarer Republik.* Historische Studien, Band 447, Helmut Castitius, Reinhard Elze, Eberhard Jäckel et al., eds. (Husum: Matthiesen, 1996), 175.

racial hygiene movements, which argued for the "cleansing" of the body of the nation, no doubt played an essential role in dehumanizing people deemed "inferior." But the socialization of German physicians, which fostered a culture of submission to the authority of one's superiors, as well as arrogant scorn for people other than German men, may have also contributed to such inhuman behavior.[18] Whether this was entirely peculiar to German physicians, however, is not entirely clear and has been the subject of scholarly debate.[19]

Assuaging the medical community's fears of lost status and safeguarding its authority cannot explain everything that needs to be explained in the often criminal behavior of physicians during the Third Reich. It was one factor among many, but one with a verifiable history that is traced in this study. The other sorts of explanations remain essentially speculative, difficult for the historian to pinpoint or document. The wholesale violations of medical ethics, the performing of hideous experiments on human beings, and the willing assistance in genocide do not seem obvious career destinations for those who practiced healing in bucolic settings. Cynical calculation of professional self-interest and the sacrifice of principles were not unique to these individuals. They typified the behavior of large portions of the German professions that made it possible for Nazism to recruit the collaboration of countless skilled, creative, and productive people. Explaining that behavior and its consequences remains one of the most pressing tasks of the historian.

---

18 see Michael H. Kater, "The Professionalization and Socialization of Physicians."

19 see Charles E. McClelland, "Modern German Doctors: A Failure of Professionalization?" in Manfred Berg and Geoffrey Cocks, eds., *Medicine and Modernity: Public Health and Medical Care in Nineteenth- and Twentieth-Century Germany* (Washington, DC: German Historical Institute and Cambridge University Press, 1996), esp. 95-97.

APPENDIX

EXCERPT OF *HANS-JÖRGELS BADEREISE*[*]

Hans-Jörgel's Spa Tour

or

Adventures on a Journey

from
Vienna to Hradisch, Luhatschowitz, Brünn, Leitomischl, Czaslau, Prag, Töplitz, Tetschen, Blasewitz, Dresden, Leipzig, Karlsbad, Marienbad, Franzensbad and back

by Water and by Land

Indispensible Handbook for Everyone who does not make the trip, but would still like to know how people eat, drink, think and speak, and one can see and hear there.

In letters to his Brother-in-Law Maxel in Feselau

Part One
Part Two

Vienna, 1842

Part One [p. 5]
And so in order to cure my injured foot and my injured humor, I asked a lot of doctors, and as it usually turns out, every one of them gave me different advice. According to the one, I should take baths in the Danube, according to the other, at the seaside, the third one said I have to take blood thickening baths, the fourth that I need to take blood thinning baths;

[*] Excerpt selected and translated by the author.

a fifth one thought it would get better on its own, but a sixth one said it's all no good, nothing can cure my ill anymore.

And so I stood there like I was lying on the Bergstrasse, and had no clue what to do, but then I came across a fellow who said, "Friend, nothing can cure you like muck!" "What?" I shout disgusted, "the muck of literature is supposed to cure my injured humor?"

"No, I can't cure your humor," he says, "for a people with sick humor they'd have to set up a special hospital [ff. p. 6] or a department in a lazaretto–I can only cure your foot, and for this I can recommend the mud baths in Franzensbad more than anything, because in cases like this and in other sicknesses, they have worked wonders."

My word, I thought, that's the punishment. All the time you couldn't stand the manure with the leatherworkers, in Leopoldstadt, in Rossau, in the alleys of Währig, in Ratysenstadt and in the other places rich in it, you were satisfied when you were only standing in it up to your ankles, and now you have it, now you're supposed to sit your whole body in it. But what could I do? That sour stuff I had to - no he didn't say anything about eating it–I was now supposed to sit in salty muck, but he assured me it would be fine.

Just think, brother-in-law, Frau Mahm, the sauerkraut maker, was prescribed a bath. She got into a dispute with her red *Schibl*, like she's always calling her husband, over a cartful of cabbage bits; her gall bladder, which even before this had to have been really big, burst–(that must have been a downpour, like in Vienna after a cloudburst in Hütteldorf, one that floods the whole beer cellar)–and the doctor prescribed her a bath.

"Ah, that's smart, cousin," she said, "so let's travel together."

"But Frau Mahm," I ask all scared, "what kind of a spa did the doctor say you should go to?"

"To … I can't remember, some hole, it's in Moravia, where you go by train–what's it called, red *Schibl*?"

"Luhatschowitz," the cousin sauerkraut maker says in such a voice, that you could see that a huge sigh was working its way from his tight chest. Just like you cry for pain and for joy, so, too, you sigh when either a great ill comes over us, or when we're freed from it. The sauerkraut maker's sigh was of a somewhat indeterminate nature, but probably it was a sigh of relief.

I let one like that out quietly, and I says to her, "But Frau Mahm, how can we go there together–Luhatschowitz and Franzensbad lie on two opposite ends of the world?

"That won't matter to you, cousin," she says, "on the railroad you go fast, it's just a little bit out of the way, and if I don't like it, I'll go right away to Karlsbad or to Franzensbad, since I can choose any one of the three."

[end page 7, begin page 8]

[page 39–in Hradisch (Hungary)]

Frau Mahm made a new acquaintance at the spring, that I could see the end of–which happened that same afternoon–right away. It was one of those unhappy adventurers that like to linger in spas. Frau Mahm told me he's a professor, somebody else who knows him better assured me that he's a steward, until a third person, who was really well informed, explained that he was a private tutor, and now wanders about as a vagabond. Frau Mahm couldn't praise him enough, what a nice and smart man he is, with the last one I had to be careful, and I didn't contradict, because there's nothing more horrible than when you try to prove a woman wrong [end page 39, begin page 40] when she thinks a man is nice and smart. You get screamed at right away for being jealous, and you, brother-in-law, can take my word that I was not jealous of him and Frau Mahm.

[p. 122]

Dr Hans-Jörgel. *)

*) Disgusting finesse! Instead of signing Dr. (servant), Hans-Jörgel signs D^{r} (Doctor)! Do others do the same thing?[1]

Endlessly remarking, the publisher.

---

[1] Translator's note: the original *fraktur* font is necessary to clarify this reference. Dr., printed in *fraktur* (or handwritten in Sütterlin), would be an abbreviation of *Diener*, or servant, whereas Hans-Jörgel supposedly made use of the Latin-script Dr for doctor. The original is as follows:
*) Entsetzlichhe Finesse! Anstatt Dr. (Diener) schreibt der Hans=Jörgel D$^{r.}$ (Doctor)! Machen es etwa Andere auch so?
Abermals bemerkend des Buchhhändlers.

[Part Two, p. 91–in Karlsbad]

We ate at the *Prince Wilhelm*, and I can assure you, Brother-in-Law, it's a guesthouse for sure like no other in the Bohemian spas as far as cheap goes. But the rooms are clean, the food is good, and if I tell you that a room costs only 30 *kreuzer* [cents] hard cash, and the portions except for the expensive dishes, only cost 15 *kreuzer* in bills, you'll have to admit that one can't find a more wonderful guesthouse.

Like Teplitz, this here [Karlsbad] is a spa where you can see that people are really sick. Mostly you see just jaundiced people, pitiful faces, what you don't notice so much when they're taking walks, because they're mixed up with so many other people, but early in the morning at the carbonated water spring and the other fountains it's really a hospital. And how wonderful the effects of these healing springs are! People drink the water for not even three weeks, and their yellow color disappears, their dull eyes get livelier, fresher, their listless gait gets more certain, more upright, in short, from this scalding hot water, that rises up from Mannsbach, where the steam rises up in thick [end page 91, begin page 92] clouds, the goddess of health laughs with her rosy red cheeks.

I couldn't help myself, Brother-in-Law, I stood in front of the spring with a feeling really moved, the kind of feeling you can't joke about. If somebody doesn't live according to a regimen, and doesn't follow exactly what his doctor prescribed him, he might, and it's already happened to some people, have to pay with his life. But there are as few doctors there as in other places, a lack of them, and because the art of medicine in Vienna has already sunken so low, that there one doctor will try to steal others' patients outright, so that they, at least a lot of them, do the coarsest, most terrible things to each other, insult and degrade each other, like a lutemaker wouldn't even do often, and so you shouldn't be surprised that it's not much better in the spas. Just think, brother-in-Law, in Karlsbad there have to be nearly twenty doctors, the way they fight for patients.

. . .

[page 93]

While the women were discussing things, I [end page 93, begin page 94] went out a bit to mingle with the spa guests, and I heard at least twenty times how somebody asked someone else: "How many cups have you drunk?" "What effect has it had?" It was really like at a fancy dress ball, where you hear nothing other than "Oh, so you're here, too!" "We've already met!" All people talked about was drinking and then about the successes, and they told about them in such a fussy way, that I started to feel sick.

The one distraction in the conversation was a death that occurred, and that for me proves how some people lose their lives in such a senseless and stupid way when they don't ask a doctor for advice, but rather take the cure on their own. He started right away with mineral water and drank twenty cups on the first day. If he had asked someone right away when he noticed it wasn't doing him any good, maybe he could have still be helped, but well, he kept on drinking until he couldn't drink any more, and then it was too late to help.

The same thing happened to a Russian a few years ago. Because he didn't speak German, but only a little Latin, the doctor prescribed him *sex pocula*–that's six cups. He looks it up in the dictionary, and finds that *poculum* means a mug. His servant had to buy him a mug, and he emptied the thing good and proper six times. Of course this really got his belly going, he got deathly ill, they called the doctor, [end page 94, begin page 95] and at first he couldn't explain the cause, until he saw the *poculum*. He was really upset he didn't notice it sooner.

When you look at the mineral deposits that collect at the spring, then it's no wonder that this year a woman couldn't be convinced to drink from it for anything in the world, because she was really sure that a crust like the one at the spring would form in her stomach or that her heart could be covered with it like the crabs or wooden figurines that people put in the spring.

But you don't have to put your heart into the spring, they turn to stone on their own, and since the woman was afraid of this, then it was a sign for me that she must have a good heart in the first place.

Frau Mahm had already made up her mind, she was staying there, and would console the woman from Rumpelsbodigen in her misfortune.[2] Then a doctor they had dug up at the spring who had treated the woman from Rumpelsbodigen says that nothing is better for her condition than mineral water, and I thanked God in my heart that I got rid of the pest.

. . .

[page 119] in Franzensbad

So, brother-in-law, here I am. My pleasant and friendly Doctor Köstler, who is employed by the government as a spa physician [*Brunnenarzt*], and because of his skill and the care he shows his patients, can be recommended to all spa guests [*Kurgäste*], he answered by request from Vienna and found me a good place to stay. ...

[page 121]

---

[2] A minor character introduced who suffered primarily from worries.

At five-thirty I have to get up, brother-in-law, and go to the spring. My doctor prescribed me the Wiesenquelle. You drink a glass, wait around for a quarter of an hour, then drink another glass, and it goes on like this for two hours.

The first time I must have made a really funny face when I drank that salty water on an empty stomach, but by the third day it got easier. I think I'll get used to it soon, it bubbles like Shampane [*Schampanier*], and nuttin' phoney, but really pure, right out of the underground pharmacy. When the sun shines you can see the pearls jumping up into the air and I'd just like to know why people, when they drink it, always turn their face away from the spring.

Is there something in us by nature that we turn our backs on those who do good for us? At least it seemed that way to me at the spring. [end page 121, begin page 122]

People come from hundreds of miles away, get healthy here again, and how few look back at the spring with gratitude, that our dear Lord God has bubble up out of the depths of the earth and its mysterious powers?

What I've seen every day, though, it's pretty dull there. Don't even think about sociability there, you don't see many people talking with each other there, except for the doctors, of whom there are only nine there, with their patients, and if somebody don't have much to say, then he's finished soon, and just mopes around.

...

So that you'll have an idea what goes on at the spring, I'll send you a picture.

One morning at the Wiesenquelle in Franzensbad I've called it, and you can see all the different types of folks who are looking for their health there. What kind of demands people make of such a spring is unbelievable. If one has a red nose, a real schnoz, then he thinks all he has to do is drink mineral water and it will shrink. Another one is a little heavy-set, and has to get thin again, if he takes the cure; the skinny ones hope to get fat again; one has too much blood, another has too little; one has excited, the other dulled nerves; one has something wrong with his head, the other in his stomach. One has a pressure on the right side, the other feels a pinch on the left. In short, what no medicine could ever heal and can't heal, a mineral spring should cure.

Doctors, when they don't know what to do with their patients, send them to a spa, and when you see people from all parts of the world, you see them with all sorts of temperaments, real and imagined sicknesses, and just imagine! Most go, if not healed, then at least healthier than they came.

Diet, getting up early, exercise in the fresh air, being away from all unpleasant business, that's for sure something you can't have so easily in the city, and when you're drinking this healing mineral water on top of that, then you can explain miracles in a natural way, and promise everyone improvement from such a cure.

What kind of people come together here, you can see in the picture. On the right is a fat one with a *paraplui*[3] who's emptying her glass in a single gulp. Her regular sort of [end page 123, begin page 124] red wraparound is in real contrast with the red velvet shawl of the lady on the left, who is having her cup presented by a servant, and is inspecting folks through her lorgnett[4].

The character of the others you can see in their faces, so what the one has too much of and too little of, and what the Wiesenquelle should give to him or replace.

I haven't taken a mud bath yet, the doctor prescribed the Francis baths first, and I have to say I'm pretty satisfied with the cleanliness and the service in the baths.

The bathhouse owner, Loimann is a very active and cultured man. The set up he's got is excellent, every bather, whether rich or poor, high or low, has his set hour at which his bath is ready. Come who may, nothing gets changed in this plan, there's one fee for everyone and everyone is treated the same. He's hired a really good bath master, and nothing fazes him. Because the old bathhouse is too small, they're building a new one, and as I see it, the bathhouse owner is sparing no costs to make it elegant and at the same time functional.

I've been here three days, and in these three days, in spite of all the compliments I was met with, I haven't talked so much, except with my charming doctor, as it looks like from this letter.

[page 125]

Wonder of wonders, brother-in-law! I took my first mud bath, and just think of my joy, my amazement, my surprise, the tension in my knee that made walking so hard, the pain was gone. Of course, only for a couple of hours, but I already felt how the mud works.

Most of all, I have to give you a description of what this kind of bath is like, and for some of my readers who maybe suffer from gout or some other malady, will know to thank me for it, since the doctor really can cure with these baths, and there's no exact description, except for the one by Doctor Köstler in a foreign paper.

---

[3] French, *parapluie*, umbrella.
[4] from French, *lorgnette*, used here to refer to small spectacles.

. . .

[page 127, in the baths]

But what a feeling, brother-in-law! Already the smell of the mud is worth something, and soon it's like when you steep herbs in wine, it's got that kind of aroma. Of course the salt eats at the roots and junk in the ground, and when the mud is pulled up and heaped in a pile, the smell is really fermented.

To find out just how salty the mud is, I licked some with my tongue. It's got an amazingly [end page 127, begin page 128] biting taste, and people whose skin is too tender can only take a bath every other day, becuase otherwise it eats at their skin.

Following my doctor's orders, I sat in there for a half an hour, and then I took the cleansing bath, and when I got out, just think of my happy surprise, since before I could hardly walk across the room without a cane and now I could go to the sofa without any effort.

Such an effect from one bath! This relief lasted an hour, and it gets better with each bath. Right away, I felt grateful to my Doctor Flechner in Vienna, who had sent me to Franzensbad, and even if I limp for the rest of my life so much that sensitive reviewers will rebuke me for this alone, because they don't know anything else other than that I limp, what one guy does most of all, him with his redhead–but pfui, dear Hans-Jörgel, if some worthless street kid throws crap at you, you'll duck and hit him with crap -- well that just slipped out because it's so funny when a redhead rebukes another guy because he limps.

When I get out of the bath, I hugged the bathhouse owner with joy, and I told him: friend, they should make gold out of this mud.

I then found out that odd cures have been done in Franzenbad. People that had to be [end page 128, begin page 129] carried into the bath or who were on crutches were dancing at the last gala ball. It really happened, brother-in-law!

But I won't dance, my dear brother-in-law, because I was at the gala ball and said: once, and never again.

A small group of real snobs found their way in there, who made the others sick, they didn't look at anybody or talk with anybody, and on top of that, they disgussed the others who were talking. But when they needed somebody for a quadrill, they were happy if one, and only one, would dance, no matter how he looked, but still everyone thanked them for the *robot* work![5]

---

[5] *Robottarbeit*, an Austrian reference to compulsory labor which peasants were required to perform for their lords.

Everybody pays the same, and then ten or twelve foolish Gretls and bellies[6] all full-of-themselves think they're beautiful, and when you've listened to their discourse, on my word, only the stupid poodle girlies in Vienna can babble so stupidly.

Among other people, I've got to know a bunch of poets here, that is, by sight at least, the ones that are here. I was really curious about Heinrich Laube, because he complains so much about Austria, then crawls back to us and we're so nice and let him crawl. And then the famous Raupach is here. The old man is really sick [end page 129, begin p. 130] and you can see it, he looks real terrible and he doesn't talk with anyone and makes faces as if he wanted to eat the whole world alive. By my word, I would have imagined the poet of the black market differently. [I also met] two Barons Platt from Hannover ... a couple of really sweet people, and have learned more than how many branches their family tree has or how many cows they have standing in the stall. ... [p. 131] I got used to the idea here, brother in law, that with people like that the best thing you can do is act is if they didn't exist at all.

. . .

[An Englishman] came from America to take the baths, and when he got here he got orders to go directly to East India. He has a kind of rash all over his body, and because the baths do him so much good he sits in there for three hours.

On his body, the rash has healed, but not in his face, and then he gets the unfortunate idea of sticking his head into the mud.

He does it right, but right away his eyes started to burn so much that he had to come right up again. He wanted to rub his eyes, but forgot or didn't see that his hands were full of mud, and then he rubs the salt into his eyes good and proper.

Now he starts to cry for help, and the mud runs into his mouth, burns his tongue, and after he spat for a while, he had to call for help.

The bath attendant didn't hear it right away, and finally notices the spectacle, throws the door open and is startled to see the poor fellow black as coal.

[page 142]

This is the last letter that you'll get from Franzensbad. The mud, or like one should really say, the moor balsam, fixed me up really well, and not just me, but everyone who bathed there are unanimous in their praise of all the apparently miraculous effects that one sees from day to day. I'd

---

[6] The original, *Batschen*, in Austrian vernacular of the period could refer either to house slippers (as it can today), or to bellies, also in an oblique reference to women with an inference to pregnancy.

just like to know why so few Viennese come to Franzensbad? [end page 142, begin page 143]

If I wrote you in my previous letter what can be criticized here, then I have to write what should be praised. Most of all, that's the hospital for poor sick people from all nations, which is supported by small contributions by spa guests, and where Doctor Köstler is the Ordinarius. The sick are provided everything they need and treated in such a humane way as if they were cavaliers. The bathhouse owner Loimann donated over 6,000 baths in three years to the hospital for free, and when I think how many poor people had baths in his bathhouse for free, well then such a fine act of generosity and humanity deserves to be publicly recognized.

The merchant Hecht deserves similar recognition, who has the francise for sending bottled mineral water. He sends several thousand jugs a year for free to hospitals and to doctors to give to the poor, and it makes me glad to see that the sun of charity that shines from Vienna over the entire Empire, and warms hearts everywhere and ispires people to good works.

[page 145]

My brother-in-law should know, that Jean Paul is my favorite writer, and I know some of his things by heart, although I haven't copied whole parts like others have. And besides, it doesn't bather me at all, because it's such a real treasure that one can never totally exploit. In one page he says as much as others do in a whole book.

. . .

Hans-Jörgel from Gumpoldskirchen

BIBLIOGRAPHY

Archival Sources

Stadtarchiv Baden-Baden:

20-1-537, Diener und Dienste, Dienstanweisungen für das Personal der Kurverwaltung.

20-7-1, Promenadeordnung. 1873+

20-13-1, Auswärtige Presse, Remunerations-Bewilligungen von Herrn Damance, 1873-1880

20-13-3, Friedrichsbad-Broschüren. 1878

20-13-4, Werbung während der Choleraepidemie, 1884

20-13-5, Badeblatt. 1891+, Kurkomittee.

20-13-6, Presseangelegenheiten 1891-1903.

20-13-8, Herstellung von Führern, Reklameplakate, Prospekte, Umgebungskarten, Klischees, etc., 1893.

20-13-9, Auswärtige Presse, Von Herrn Redakteur Harder geschriebenen Artikel, zur Versendung in auswärtigen Zeitungen.

20-13-12, Herausgabe des Neuen Prospectes, 1897

20-13-14, Auswärtige Presse: Korrespondenzen des Herrn St?? in auswärtige Zeitungen, 1900+

20-13-16, Werbung, Allgemein, 1904-1909

20-13-17, Verkehrsbüro, Propaganda Beitrag des Ministeriums des Innern, 1910+

20-13-18, Artikel der Frankfurter Zeitung von Herrn Professor Dr. Stern, 1910

20-13-19, Verkehrsbureau: Propaganda und Festschrift, 1912+

20-13-20, Unabhängigkeit von der Presse, 1913.

20-14-1, Einrichtung und Betrieb des Spielsaals im Kurhaus, 1872-1914

20-16-8, Deutsches Zentralkomitee für ärztliche Studienreisen, 1909+, Kurkomitee

20-16-3, Verein der Kurorte und Mineralquellen-Interessenten. 1894+. Kurkomitee

20-16-15, Badischer Landesverband zur Erhebung des Fremdenverkehrs. 1906-13

20-17-152, Gestaltung der Kurverwaltung, 1872

20-17-153, Rechenschaftsberichte der Kurverwltungskasse, 1877+

20-17-155, Curörtliche Verhältnisse von Baden Baden, 1877-1888
25-1-23, Bezirksamt, Medicin-Anstalten, 1870
25-1-24, Medizinalwesen, 1889.

26-15-64, Promenadenbuden. Verpachtung, Offenhaltung u. Schliessung. 1901-27. Stadtrat, Kursachen.
26-15-184, Subventionierung Baden-Iffezheimer Pferderennen, Stadtrat, Kursachen. 1906-18
26-29-173, Verkehrswesen: Prospekt von Baden-Baden, 1906

Badisches Generallandesarchiv Karlsruhe:
Abteilung 195, Akten Baden-Baden Stadt
(a combined archival category, which combines materials from various city and state archival classifications. Origins of the documents noted when necessary with the following abbreviations in use: BAKom= Bäderkomission; MdI= Ministerium des Innern; Geh.Rat= Geheimer Staatsrat).
Nr. 294, 1805-1808. Bestellung einer Badkomission und deren Wirksamkeit zur Emporbringung des Bades (Oberamt).
Nr. 964. 1801-1805. Emporbringung der warmen Bäder. Enthält: Bemerkungen des Hof- und Reg.Rats. Poßelt, die Bäder auch hinsichtlich der inneren Verbesserungen und äußeren Verschönerungen, v. 1801. (Amtsakten)
Nr. 965, 1801-1805. Zur Emporbringung des Badener Bades getroffenen Anstalten. (Hofrat).
Nr. 966-968, 1804-1822. Zur Emporbringung der Bäder von seiten der Landesherrschaft getroffenenen Vorkehrungen (Finanzdepartement)
Nr. 1031, 1805. Das Bad und damit in Verbindung stehende Gegenstände.
Nr. 1060. 1805-1807. Badberichte, Berichterstattungen über den Fremdenverkehr im Bade.
Nr. 1077, 1806. Während der Anwesenheit der Badkommission abgehaltene Protokolle. (Amtsakten)
Nr. 1061. 1806-1808. Oberamtsberichte über die in Baden angekommenen und wieder abgereisten Badgäste; die Badlisten
Nr. 1062, 1807. Gedruckte und handschriftliche Verzeichnisse der Kurgäste in Baden-Baden.
Nr. 1063, 1807. Die Bad-Polzeiordnung zu Baden.
Nr. 1080, 1807-1808. Akten der Bad-Direktion in Baden überschrieben: „Bad-Direktionsangelegenheiten", insbesondere die Einrichtung der Hazardspiele.

Nr. 1064. Die in Vorschlag gekomene Anstellung eines besonderen Bad- und Polizei-Komissärs. (Justizministerium)

Nr. 971, 1809, Den Kromerschen Plan über die Leitung des warmen Wassers in die verschiedenen Badhäuser der Stadt. (Amtsakten)

Nr. 1034-1037, 1809-1813. In dem Bad gemachten Einrichtungen (Geh.Rat).

Nr. 1065, 1810. Badlisten bzw. Verzeichnisse über die in Baden sich aufhaltenden Fremden (Badgäste)

Nr. 1084, 1810-1812. Anlegung eines englischen Gartens und Bassins; polizeiliche Verordnungen gegen die Beschädigung der Pflanzen, Geländeankauf. (MdI)

Nr. 972, 1811. Belohnung der Verdienste des Amtmanns Schetzler und des Ratsverwandten Georg Schneider um das Gemeindewesen, insbesondere die Badanstalten daselbst.

Nr. 1093, 1811-1823. Die englischen Anlagen bei dem Promenadehaus und die Verbindung einiger Promandewege mit demselben, sowie die Unterhaltung der Gärten, Anlagen, Alleen und Promenaden überhaupt. (MdI).

Nr. 1039, 1815-1817. Ärztliche Behandlung der armen Badegäste und die dafür ausgeworfene Belohnung (Amtsakten)

Nr. 978, 1817-1822. Verbesserung der Bäder, Errichtung eines Dampfbades, Zubereitung des Karlsbader Wassers und die Verpachtung des Dampfbades. (Amtsakten)

Nr. 979, 1817-1827. Berichte des Physikats über die beobachteten Wirkungen des Badwassers bei Krankheitsfällen; sowie die Veröffentlichungen in französischen Blättern über die Eigenschaften und Wirkungen der Heilquellen.

Nr. 988-989, 1826-1856. Die öffentlichen Badanstalten und die Generalberichte über den Kurort. Enthält u.a. Errichtung einer Badanstalten-Komission und Regulativ für diesselbe, 1835). (BAKom).

Nr. 1099, 1829-1830. Erbauung einer Kurhalle auf der Promenade. (MdI).

Nr. 1109, 1837-1839. Errichtung einer öffentlichen Badeanstalt in Baden. Auch Erbauung einer Trinkhalle. (MdI)

Nr. 1066, 1838. Denkschrift des Freiherrn Ferdinand v. Schweizer, späteren badischen Gesandten in Paris die Fremdenpolizei in Baden-Baden und die Ernennung eines Bade-Komissärs (Bäderintendanten). (MdI).

Nr, 994. 1847-1854. Aufstellung der Budgets der Badanstalten. (BAKom)

Nr. 995. 1853-1862. Die Badanstalten zu Baden, insbesondere gesundheitliche Reglement für dieselben, Zusammenstellungen über die Zahl und Art der verabreichten Bäder. (BAKom)

Nr. 1085-1087, 1810-1827. Das Dampfbad-Etablissement und was sonst auf Verbesserung oder Erweiterung desselben bezug hat. I-III, Fortsetzung s. 236/3364.

Nr. 1089, 1819-1842. Das Dampfbad, Betrieb und Einrichtung (BAKom).

Nr. 1090, 1841-1842. Errichtung eines russischen Dampfbades im Hirschwirtshaus (BAKom).

Nr. 1091-1092, 1856-1864. Das Dampfbad, insbesondere den Betrieb desselben (BAKom).

Nr. 1202, 1808. Aufsicht und Handhabung der Ordnung auf Badener Alleen und Promenaden.

Nr. 1218, 1822-1854. Spielordnung (-Reglement) für die Bank (BAKom)

Nr. 1232, 1850-1866. Herausgabe einer offiziellen Fremdenliste in der Stadt. Enthält: Zusammenstellungen der Fremden nach Nationalitäten geordnet. (BAKom)

Bestand 339: Bezirksamt/Landratsamt Baden-Baden [Regional Administration]

No. 954. Vollzug der Verordnung wegen dem Hazard Spiel, insbesondere das Verbot des Spielens hiesiger Einwohner, Handwerksburschen, Studenten und anderer Personen. 1767-1864.

No. 1200. Gemeingefährliche Bestrebungen der Sozialdemokratie; hier: Verbreitung sozialdemokratischer Druckschriften, Beschlagnahme derselben.

No. 1203. Gemeingefährliche Bestrebungen der sozialdemokratischer Partei. Hier: Vorbereitung des Verbotes sozialdemokrat. Druckschriften im Amtsbereich Baden. Darin: „Aufrufe“ and die Bevölkerung (1891), Wahlkampfaufruf zur Reichstagswahl (1887), „Volksfreund“ Nr. 15. vom 6.2. 1887, „Wähler“ (Flugblatt, 18.1.1887, herausgegeben von Adolf Yeck.). 1880-1890.

No. 1210. Sozialdemokratische Umtriebe des Dr. med. Lazar Wischnewsky aus Tageroy (Rußland). 1888-1891.

No. 1228. Vollzug der Verordnung über die Bücherzensur, Verkauf von Büchern, Anlegung von Druckereien, Lehr- und Leihbibliotheken; Herausgabe von Zeitungen und Volkskalendern, Verkauf von Druckschriften. 1819, 1832-88.

No. 1229. Druck, Verlag und Zensur der dahier erscheinenden Badezeitung, des Tag-, Unterhaltungs- und Wochenblattes; Aufstellung der Zensoren. 1819-21, 1841-45.

No. 1236. Statistik der Wohltätigkeits- und Krankenanstalten, Orden und Kongregationen, Waisenhäuser, Erziehungsanstalten.
No. 1256. Verordnung und deren Vollzug betr. 1. Bestimmung der Badeplätze. 1828-1838.
No. 1258. Verordnungen und Aufsicht über Reisende, Wallfahrer, Künstler, Landstreicher u.a.; Ausfertigung und Kontrolle der Papiere und Bücher. 1804-1849
No. 1270. Verordnungen und Aufsicht über Reisende, Wallfahrer, Künstler, Landstreicher u.a.; Ausfertigung und Kontrolle der Papiere und Bücher. 1850-1863
No. 1275. Verordnungen und Vorschriften wegen Abhaltung und Beaufsichtigung der öffentlichen Tanzbelustigungen, Handhabung der Sonntagsfeier, Besuch der Wirtshäuser und Tanzböden durch Sonntagsschüber, Maßregeln gegen übermäßiges Zechen und Schwelgereien, ferner die weltliche Feier der Kirchweih. 1708-1715; 1747; 1766-78; 1805, 1814, 1826-1865
No. 1279. Verordnungen und Vorschriften betr. Handhabung der Polizeistunde, Maßregeln gegen das Nachschwärmen, Übersitzen in den Wirtschaften, Bekämpfung der Trunksucht. 1795; 1824-39; 1856-60.
No. 1338. Ausübung der Heilkunde durch nicht approbierte Personen; hier Rudolf Blitz und die „Gesellschaft zur Vorbeugung der Krankheiten in der menschlichen Rasse."
No. 1344. Handhabung der öffentlichen Sicherheit und Ordnung bei den Pferderennen zu Iffezheim. 1858-1873; 1883-1893.
No. 1364. Vorschriften wegen Aufnahme in das Armenbad oder Solbad und Bestimmung der Kostpreise. 1828-1868.
No. 1377. Vorschriften über Besetzung und Verwaltung der Stelle des Bezirksarztes, Personal- und Dienstverhältnisse der Ärzte und Dienstinstruktionen. 1772-78; 1805; 1815-1878.
No. 1421. Beschwerden über Dirnen, 1907-1913.
No. 1422. Überwachen der Dirnen. 1916-1918.
No. 1446. Prüfung, Verpflichtung und Niederlassung der Ärzte, 1875-1886

Newspapers, Periodicals

Morgenblatt für Gebildete Stände.
Morgenblatt für Gebildete Leser.
Badeblatt. Baden-Baden, 1808-1913.
Illustriertes Bade-Blatt 14, nos. 9-19 (April-August, 1892).

Balneologische Zeitung. Correspondenzblatt der deutschen Gesellschaft für Hydrologie 1, nos. 1-12 (January 1, 1855-December 17, 1855) and 2, nos. 1-7 (February 25, 1856-November 12, 1856).

Published Sources

AEIOU, Das Kulturinformationssystem des Bundesministerium für Bildung, Wissenschaft und Kultur [Austria], at http://www.aeiou.at/aeiou.encyclop.t/t950672.htm, accessed July 14, 2004.

Ahrlé, Ferry. *Baden-Baden: Zauber d. Fassaden: Impressionen.* Baden-Baden: Wesel, 1975.

Albisetti, James, Charles E. McClelland and R. Steven Turner. "Science in Germany." *Osiris* 2nd Series, 5. Issue Science in Germany: The Intersection of Institutional and Intellectual Issues (1999): 285-304.

Altendorf, Ewald. *Die Badereise.* Berlin: Hesperus Verlag, 1912.

Amelung, W. "Zur Geschichte der Bäder- und Klimaheilkunde." In Amelung, W. and G. Hildebrandt, eds. *Balneologie und medizinische Klimatologie.* 3rd revised edition. Berlin, Heidelberg: Springer Verlag, 1986.

Aquae. Baden-Baden: Der Arbeitskreis für Stadtgeschichte der Stadt Baden-Baden, 1986

Bad Boll, 1595-1995: vom herzoglichen Wunderbad zum Kurort. Weissenhorn: A.H. Konrad, 1995.

Badeärztlicher Verein Baden-Baden. *So heilt Baden-Baden. Eine medizin.-balneolog. Darstellung.* Uelzen, Medizinisch-Literarischer Verl., 1966.

Baden-Baden damals: alte Photographien erzählen ein Stück Stadtgeschichte: 1860-1910. Konstanz: Stadler, 1978.

Bäder-Almanach. Mittheilungen aus den Bädern, Luftcurorten und Heilanstalten in Deutschland, Oesterreich, Schweiz und der angrenzenden Gebiete für Aerzte und Heilbedürftige. Frankfurt a.M., Berlin: Rudolf Mosse, 1882.

Bäder-Handbuch. Edited by the Allgemeiner Deutscher Bäderverband. Breslau: Allgemeine Deutsche Bäderzeitung, 1916.

Bajohr, Frank. *"Unser Hotel ist judenfrei." Bäder-Antisemitismus im 19. und 20. Jahrhundert.* Frankfurt am Main: Fischer Taschenbuchverlag, 2003.

Balling, F.A. *Die Heilquellen und Bäder zu Kissingen für Kurgäste.* 1850.

Barnett, L. Margaret. review of *Making Medicine Scientific: John Burdon Sanderson and the Culture of Victorian Science* by Terrie M. Romano,

Journal of the American Medical Association 289 (June 25, 2003): 3312.

Baumgärtner, J., Hoffmann, Hugo von, et al. *Baden-Baden und seine Kurmittel. Im Auftrage des Badener ärztlichen Vereins bearbeitet.* Baden-Baden, Verlag von C. Wild's Hofbuchhandlung, 1886.

Beattie, William. *Journal of a Residence in Germany, Written during a Professional Attendance on Their Royal Highnesses the Duke and Duchess of Clarence, (Their Most Gracious Majesties) during Their Visits to the Courts of that Countrz in 1822, 1825 & 1826.* London: Longman, Rees, Ohme, Brown & Green, 1831.

Benaroyo, Lazare. "Rudolf Virchow and the Scientific Approach to Medicine,." *Endeavour* 22, no. 3 (1998).

Benedict, Barbara M. "Consumptive Communities: Commodifying Nature in Spa Society." *The Eighteenth Century* 36, no. 3 (1995): 203-219.

Benzler, A. *Das Ostseebad Zoppot bei Danzig. Zur Orientierung für Badegäste.* Danzig, 1882.

Berg, Manfred and Cocks, Geoffrey, ed. *Medicine and Modernity: Public Health and Medical Care in Nineteenth- and Twentieth-Century Germany.* New York: Cambridge U. Pr., 1997. 244 pp.

Berl, Heinrich. *Baden-Baden im Zeitalter der Romantik: die literarische und musikalische Romantik des neunzehnten Jahrhunderts.* Baden-Baden: Willy Schmidt, 1981.

Berzelius, Jacob. *Reiseerinnerungen aus Deutschland.* Gisbert Klingemann, ed. Berlin: Verlag Chemie, 1948.

Beschreibung der Fresken in der Neuen Trinkhalle zu Baden. 3rd expanded edition. Baden: Bureau der Badzeitung von G. Muhl [ca. 1850].

Bismarck, Otto von. *Fürst Bismarcks Briefe an seine Braut und Gattin,* Fürst Herbert Bismarck, ed. Stuttgart: J.G. Cotta'sche Buchhandlung Nachfolger, 1900.

—. *Gedanken und Erinnerungen.* Neue Ausgabe, 3 vols. Stuttgart and Berlin: J.G. Cotta'sche Buchhandlung Nachfolger, 1921.

Bitz, Mathias. *Badewesen in Südwestdeutschland 1550 bis 1840. Zum Wandel von Gesellschaft und Architektur.* Idstein: Schultz-Kirchner Verlag, 1989.

Blackbourn, David and Richard J. Evans, eds. *The German Bourgeoisie. Essays on the Social History of the German Middle Class from the Late Eighteenth Century to the Early Twentieth Century.* London and New York: Routledge, 1991.

Blackbourn, David. "Taking the Waters:' Meeting Places of the Fashionable World." in Martin H. Geyer and Johannes Paulmann, eds.,

The Mechanics of Internationalism. Culture, Society and Politics from the 1840s to the First World War. Oxford, New York: Oxford University Press, 2001, 435-457.

—. *The Long Nineteenth Century: A History of Germany, 1780-1918.* New York: Oxford University Press, 1998.

Blanchard, Ian, ed. *Labor and Leisure in Historical Perspective, Thirteenth to Twentieth Centuries.* Stuttgart: F. Steiner, 1994. 198 pp.

Blecker, Johanna. "Biedermeyermedizin: Medizin der Biedermeyer? 1830-1850." *Medizinhistorisches Journal* 23 (1988) 5-22.

—. Between Romantic and Scientific Medicine: Johann Lukas Schoenlein and the Natural History School 1825-1845. *Clio Medica* 1983 18(1-4): 191-202.

—. *Die Naturhistorische Schule 1825-1845: Ein Beitrag zur Geschichte der Klinischen Medizin in Deutschland.* New York: Gustav Fischer, 1981. 175 pp.

Bleymehl-Eiler, Martina. "Das Paradies der Kurgäste'–Die Bäder Wiesbaden, Langenschwalbach und Schlangenbad im 17. und 18. Jahrhundert." In: Michael Matheus, ed., *Badeorte und Bäderreisen in Antike, Mittelalter und Neuzeit.* Mainzer Vorträge 5. Stuttgart: Institut für Geschichtliche Landeskunde and der Universität Mainz/Fritz Steiner Verlag, 2001.

Blumenfeld, F., Fresenius, H., et al. *Ärztliche Festschrift zur Eröffnung des Städitschen Kaiser Friedrich Bades in Wiesbaden.* Wiesbaden, Verlag von J.F. Bergmann, 1913.

Borocz, Jozsef. "Travel-Capitalism: the Structure of Europe and the Advent of the Tourist." *Comparative Studies in Society and History.* 1992 34(4): 708-741.

Böttcher, J.E. *Der Seebade-Ort Zoppot bei Danzig in geschichtlicher, topographischer, statistischer, naturwissenschaftlicher und socialer Hinsicht, sein Sagenkreis und seine Wirksamkeit als Santiäts-Anstalt.* Danzig, 1842.

Böttcher, Karl. *Karlsbader Schlendertage. Bilder aus dem Saisonsleben.* Feller's Bade- und Reiesebibliothek No. 9. Karlsbad and Nice: Verlag von Hans Feller, 1884.

Braun, Rudolf. "Zur Professionalisierung des Ärztestandes in der Schweiz," in *Bildungsbürgertum im 19. Jahrhundert*, ed. Werner Conze and Jürgen Kocka, 332-357. Industrielle Welt. Schriftenreihe des Arbeitskreises für moderne Sozialgeschichte, ed. Werner Conze, No. 38. Klett-Cotta, 1985.

Broman, Thomas H. *The Transformation of German Academic Medicine, 1750-1820.* Cambridge: Cambridge University Press, 1996.

Broman, Thomas. "Rethinking Professionalization: Theory, Practice and Professional Ideology in Eighteenth Century German Medicine" *Journal of Modern History* 67, no. 4 (Dec. 1995).

—. "University Reform in Medical Thought at the End of the Eighteenth Century." *Osiris*, 2nd Series 5, Issue Science in Germany: The Intersection of Institutional and Intellectual Issues (1989): 36-53.

Brugelmann, Jan. Observations on the Process of Medicalization in Germany, 1770-1830, based on Medical Topographies. *Historical Reflections* 1982 9(1-2): 131-149.

Brüggemann, Wolfgang, ed. *Kneipptherapie: ein bewährtes Naturheilverfahren*. 2nd revised edition. Berlin, Heidelberg: Springer Verlag, 1986.

Budde, Gunilla-Friederike. *Auf dem Weg ins Bürgerleben. Kindheit und Erziehung in deutschen und englischen Bürgerfamilien, 1840-1914*. Vol. 6, *Bürgertum: Beiträge zur europäischen Gesellschaftsgeschichte*, Wolfgang Mager, Klaus Schreiner et al., eds. Göttingen: Vanderhoeck & Ruprecht, 1994.

Bueltzingsloewen, Isabelle von. "Confessionnalisation et medicalisation des soins aux malades au XIXe siècle: Essai de Reflexion á partir des cas allemand et français. [Confessionalization and medicalization in the care of the sick during the 19th century: a reflective essay based on German and French cases]. *Revue d'Histoire Moderne et Contemporaine* 1996 43(4): 632-651.

—. "Naissance de la Clinique Allemande." [Birth of the German clinic]. *Gesnerus* 1994 51(3-4): 183-199.

Burgess, J. Peter. *Meaning and Science in Weimar–Crisis and the Cultural Foundations of Reason.* European University Institute, Florence, Department of History and Civilization Working Paper HEC No. 2000/8. San Domenico: Badia Fisolana, 2000.

Burke, Peter. "The Invention of Leisure in Early Modern Europe." *Past & Present* 1995 (146): 136-150.

Burleigh, Michael. *Ethics and Extermination: Reflections on Nazi Genocide*. New York: Cambridge University Press, 1997.

Bynum, W. F. *Science and the Practice of Medicine in the Nineteenth Century*. New York: Cambridge U. Pr., 1994. 283 pp.

Cantor, D. Phyllis Hembry (edited and completed by Leonard W. Cowie and Evelyn E. Cowie), "British Spas from 1815 to the Present: A Social History." *Social History of Medicine : the Journal of the Society for the Social History of Medicine*. Vol. 11, No. 2 (1998) p. 349.

Cayleff, Susan E. Roy Porter (ed.). "The Medical History of Waters and Spas." *Bulletin of the History of Medicine*. Vol. 66, No. 1, pp. 151-152.

Chambers, Thomas A. *Drinking the Waters. Creating an American Leisure Class at Nineteenth-Century Mineral Springs.* Washington and London: Smithsonian Institution Press, 2002.

Chèzy, Wilhelm von. *Rundgemälde von Baden-Baden, seinen Nähern und fernern Umgebungen. Ein Taschenbuch für Kurgäste und Reisende.* Karlsruhe and Baden, Marx'sche Buch- und Kunsthandlung, 1835.

Cocks, Geoffrey and Konrad H. Jarausch, eds. *German Professions, 1850-1950.* New York, Oxford: Oxford University Press, 1990.

Cocks, Geoffrey. *Treating Mind and Body: Essays in the History of Science, Professions, and Society under Extreme Conditions.* New Brunswick, NJ: Transaction Publishers, 1998.

Cole, Richard G. "In Search of a New Mentality: the Interface of Academic and Popular Medicine in the Sixteenth Century." *Journal of Popular Culture* 1993 26(4): 155-172.

Compton, Michael T. "The Association of Hygieia with Asklepios in Graeco-Roman Asklepieion Medicine." *Journal of the History of Medicine and Allied Sciences* 57, no 3 (2002): 312-329.

Conze, Werner and Jürgen Kocka, et al. eds., *Bildungbürgertum im 19. Jahrhundert.* 4 volumes. Stuttgart: Klett-Cotta, 1985-92.

Corbin, Alain. *The Lure of the Sea: The Discovery of the Seaside in the Western World, 1750-1840.* Jocelyn Phelps, transl. Berkeley: University of California Press, 1994.

Corpus Inscriptionum Latinarum, 6.15258.

Crighton, James. "Some Descriptions of Schizophrenia-like Illness in the German Literature of the Early Nineteenth Century." *History of Psychiatry* 1996 7(1): 31-54.

Daum, Andreas W. *Wissenschaftspopularisierung im 19. Jahrhundert: Bürgerliche Kultur, naturwissenschaftliche Bildung und die deutsche Öffentlichkeit, 1848-1914.* Munich: Oldenbourg, 1998.

de la Roi-Frey, Karin. Frauenleben *im Biedermeier. Berühmte Besucherinnen bei Justinus Kerner in Weinsberg.* Leinfelden-Echterdingen: DRW-Verlag, 1998.

De Vierville, Jonathan Paul. *American Healing Waters: A Chronology (1513-1946) and Historical Survey of America's Major Springs, Spas, and Health Resorts Including a Review of Their Medicinal Virtues, Therapeutic Methods, and Health Care Practices* (Vols. I and II). Ph.D. Dissertation, The University of Texas at Austin, 1992

Decken-Himmelreich, Leopold von der. *Priessnitz und die Wasserkur: Aertze und Allopathie wissenschaftlich konfrontirt.* Breslau: 1845.

Dettbarn-Reggentin, Jürgen. *Strandbad Wannsee. Badegeschichte aus achtzig Jahren.* Berlin: Nishen, 1987.

Deutschlands Heilquellen und Bäder. Herausgegeben vom Kaiserlichen Gesundheits-Amt zu Berlin. Berlin: Oswald Seehagen's Verlag (Martin Hoefer), 1900.

Die Seebadeanstalt zu Zoppot bei Danzig. Danzig: J.C. Albertische Buch- und Kunsthandlung, 1823.

Die wichtigsten Bäder Europa's. Zur Empfehlung der Bäder für Gesunde und Kranke. Berlin, 1820.

Dinges, Martin, ed. *Medizinkritische Bewegungen im Deutschen Reich (ca. 1870–ca. 1933)*. MedGG Beihefte 9. Stuttgart: Steiner Verlag, 1996.

Dostoevsky, Fyodor. *The Player*. In: *Gesammelte Werke in Zwanzig Bänden*. Gerhard Dudek and Michael Wegner, eds. *Der Spieler. Späte Prosa*. Trans. from Russian into German by Werner Creutziger, ed. Gerhard Dudek. Berlin and Weimar: Aufbau-Verlag, 1990.

Draheim, Joachim. Reimann, Ute, eds. *Johannes Brahms in den Bädern Baden- Baden, Wiesbaden, Bad Ischl, Karlsbad*. Baden-Baden: Die Stadt, Baden-Baden, 1997.

Drees, Annette. *Die Ärzte auf dem Weg zu Prestige und Wohlstand. Sozialgeschichte der württembergischen Ärzte im 19. Jahrhundert*. Münster: Coppenrath, 1988.

Droste-Hülshoff, I. von. *Ems und seine Heilquellen für Bade- und Brunnengäste*. Münster: Theissingsche Buchhandlung, 1831.

Ebhardt, Franz. Der gute Ton in allen Lebenslagen. Ein Handbuch für den Verkehr in der Familie, in der Gesellschaft und im öffentlichen Leben. Fifteenth edition. Leipzig and Berlin: Julius Klinkhardt, [ca. 1900].

Ebhardt, Franz. *Der Gute Ton in allen Lebenslagen*. Leipzig and Berlin: Verlag von Julius Klinkhardt, 1900.

Ebstein, Erich, ed. *Ärzte-Memoiren aus vier Jahrhunderten*. Berlin: Verlag von Julius Springer, 1923.

Eckhart, Wolfgang U. *Geschichte der Medizin*, 3rd revised edition. Berlin: Springer Verlag, 1998.

—. "Die wachsende Nervösität underer Zeit.' Medizin und Kultur um 1900 am Beispiel einer Modekrankheit." In G. Hübinger, R. v. Bruch, F.W. Graf, eds., *Kultur und Kulturwissenschaften um 1900. Vol. II, Idealismus und Positivismus*. Stuttgart: Steiner Verlag, 1997, 207-226.

Eder, Ernst Gerhard. *Bade- und Schwimmkultur in Wien. Sozialhistorische und kulturanthropologische Untersuchungen*. Kulturstudien Bibliothek der Kulturgeschichte vol. 25, Hubert Christian Ehalt and Helmut Konrad eds. Vienna: Böhlau Verlag, 1995.

Edward Shorter, "Private Clinics in Central Europe, 1850-1933." *Social History of Medicine* 1990 3(2): 159-195.

Effern, Renate. *Der Dreiköpfige Adler. Rußland zu Gast in Baden-Baden.* Baden-Baden: Nomos, 1997.

Eghegian, Greg. *Making Security Social: Disability, Insurance, and the Birth of the Social Entitlement State in Germany.* Ann Arbor: University of Michigan Press, 2000.

Eliav, Yaron Z. "The Roman Bath as a Jewish Institution: Another Look at the Encounter between Judaism and the Greco-Roman Culture." *Journal for the Study of Judaism*, 31, no. 4 (November 2000): 416-454.

Elkeles, Barbara. "Das Krankenhaus um die Wende vom 19. zum 20. Jahrhundert aus der Sicht seiner Patienten. *Historia Hospitalium* 1986-88 17: 89-105.

Evans, Richard J. "Prostitution, State and Society in Imperial Germany." *Past and Present* 70 (February, 1976).

Ewich, Otto. *Praktisches Handbuch über die vorzüglichsten Heilquellen und Kurorte, für Aerzte und Badereisende.* Berlin: August Hirschwald, 1862.

Ewich, Otto. *Rationelle Balneologie. Praktisches Handbuch über die vorzüglichsten Heilquellen und Curorte für Aerzte und Badereisende.* Berlin: Verlag von August Hirschwald, 1862.

Fagan, Garrett G. *Bathing in Public in the Roman World.* Ann Arbor: University of Michigan Press, 1999.

Fehr, Götz and Gerhart Egger, eds. *Große Welt reist ins Bad, 1800-1914.* Passau: Passavia, 1981.

Fields, Wayne. "The Double Life of Hot Springs." *American Heritage.* Vol. 42, No. 2, (April, 1991) p. 106.

Fischer, Bernhard. *Der Badische Hof 1807-1830. Cottas Hotel in Baden-Baden*. Marbacher Magazin, No. 79/1997. Marbach am Neckar: Deutsche Schillergesellschaft, 1997.

Fontane, Theodor. "Die Sommerfrischen." In: *Von Zwanzig bis Dreissig. Autobiographisches Nebst anderen selbstbiographischen Zeugnissen.* [Originally published 1898] in *Theodor Fontane, Sämtliche Werke*, Kurt Schreinert and Jutta Neuendorff-Fürstenau, eds. Munich: Nymphenburger Verlagshandlung, 1967.

Foucault, Michel. *The Birth of the Clinic: An Archaeology of Medical Perception*. New York, 1973.

Frech, Karl. *Entwurf für das Neue Dampfbad in Baden-Baden mit begefügtem Grundrisse.* Baden: Scotyniovsky'sche Buchdruckerei, 1861.

—. *Der Kurort Baden-Baden, Ein Beitrag zur Geschichte des heutigen Badewesens* (Karlsruhe: Chr. Fr. Müller'sche Hofbuchhandlung, 1870.

—. *Die russischen Thermaldampfbäder in Baden-Baden. Anleitung zum Gebrauch derselben sowie der russischen Bäder überhaupt.* Lahr: Verlag von M. Schnauenberg & C., 1862.

Freidson, Eliot. *Profession of Medicine. A Study in the Sociology of Applied Knowledge.* New York: Dodd, Mead, 1975.

Frevert, Ute. "Professional Medicine and the Working Classes in Imperial Germany," in *Journal of Contemporary History* 20, no. 4 (October 1984): 637-658.

Frey, A. and F. Heiligenthal. *Die Heissen Luft- und Dampfbäder in Baden-Baden. Experimentelle Studie über ihre Wirkung und Anwendung.* Leipzig: Verlag von F.C.W. Vogel, 1881.

Frey, A., ed. *Der Schwarzwald und seine Kurorte.* Baden-Baden: Verlag von D.R. Marx, Hof-Buchhandlung (W.F. Gneisig), 1891.

Frey, A., ed. *Der Schwarzwald und seine Kurorte.* Baden-Baden. 1891.

Frey, Manuel. *Der reinliche Bürger*, Kritische Studien zur Geschichtswissenschaft vol. 119, Helmut Berding, Jürgen Kocka, Hans-Peter Ullmann, Hans-Ulrich Wehler, eds. Göttingen: Vanderhoeck & Ruprecht, 1996.

Friedlander, Henry. *The Origins of Nazi Genocide: From Euthanasia to the Final Solution.* Chapel Hill: University of North Carolina Press, 1995.

Das Friedrichbad in Baden-Baden. Beschreibung des Baues und Anleitung zum Gebrauche der Bäder und der Trinkkur, nebst Badeordnung. Baden-Baden, D.M. Marx'sche Hofbuchhandlung, 1878.

Fromherz, Albert. *Baden-Baden zur Franzosenzeit. Skizzen aus dem Badeleben vor fünfzig Jahren.* Edited and with an introduction by Karl Hauck. Baden-Baden: Peter Weber, 1905.

Frommel, Carl Ludwig. *Baden-Baden.* folded leaf of plates : ill. ; 18 cm. Reprint. Originally published: Baden und seine Umgebungen in malerischen Ansichten /von Professor Frommel ; mit einer historisch-topographischen Beschreibung von Hofrath Schreiber. Dortmund: Harenberg, 1979.

Fuhs, Burkhard. *Mondäne Orte einer Vornehmen Gesellschaft. Kultur und Geschichte der Kurstädte 1700-1900.* Historische Texte und Studien, vol. 13. Hildesheim, Zürich, New York: Olms Verlag, 1992.

Gall, Lothar. *Bürgertum in Deutschland.* Berlin: Siedler, 1989.

Gall, Lothar, ed. *Stadt und Bürgertum im 19. Jahrhundert.* Munich: Oldenbourg, 1990.

Gall, Lothar. *Von der ständischen zur bürgerlichen Gesellschaft,* (Munich: Oldenbourg, 1993), 13-14.

Genth, D.E.A. *Untersuchungen über den Einfluß des Wassertrinkens auf den Stoffwechsel.* Wiesbaden, 1856.

Geuss, Raymond. "Kultur, Bildung, Geist." *History & Theory* 35, no. 3 (1996): 151-163.

Gideon, Sigfried. *Geschichte des Bades.* Hamburg: Europäische Verlagsanstalt, 1988.

Göckenjan, Gerd. „Wandlungen im Selbstbild des Arztes." in *Medizin, Mensch und Gesellschaft* 13 (1988)

Goethert, Klaus-Peter. "Badekultur, Badeorte, Bäderreise in den gallischen Provinzen," in Michael Matheus, ed., *Badeorte und Bäderreisen in Antike, Mittelalter und Neuzeit.* Mainzer Vorträge 5. Stuttgart: Institut für Geschichtliche Landeskunde and der Universität Mainz/Fritz Steiner Verlag, 2001.

Götz, Aly, Peter Chroust and Christian Pross. *Cleansing the Fatherland: Nazi Medicine and Racial Hygiene.* Baltimore: Johns Hopkins University Press, 1994.

Goubert, Jean-Pierre. *The Conquest of Water.* [Original: Conquête de l'eau, translated by Andrew Wilson]. Princeton: Princeton University press, 1989.

Gregory, Frederick. "Regulative Therapeutics in the German Romantic Era: The Contribution of Jakob Friedrich Fries (1773-1843)." *Clio Medica* 1983 18(1-4): 179-190.

Grosse Welt reist ins Bad, 1800-1914 : Baden bei Wien, Badgastein, Bad Ischl, Franzensbad, Karlsbad, Marienbad, Teplitz : eine Ausstellung des Adalbert Stifter Vereins, München in Zusammenarbeit mit dem Österreichischen Museum für Angewandte Kunst, Wien : Schloss Grafenegg bei Krems, Niederösterreich, vom 10. Mai bis 3.November 1980 Wien: Österreichisches Museum für Angewandte Kunst, 1980.

Grün, Caroline. *Kurorte in Bayern under besonderer Berücksichtigung des Einflusses der Sozialversicherungsträger.* Dr.oec.publ. dissertation, Ludwig-Maximilians-Universität München, 1994.

Guinot, Eugen. *Ein Sommer in Baden-Baden.* Leipzig: Verlagsbuchhandlung von J.J. Weber, 1858.

Guthmann, Alfred. *Wie soll der gesunde und kranke Kurgast im Ostseebade leben? Ein Wegweiser für die Badegäste der Ostsee.* Berlin: Hugo Steinitz, 1905.

Haebler, Rolf Gustav. *Geschcihte der Stadt und des Kurortes Baden-Baden.* 2 volumes, Second Edition. Baden-Baden: Verlag Dr. Willy Schmidt, 1969.

Hahn, Gernot von and Hans-Kaspar von Schönfels. *Wunderbares Wasser. Von der heilsamen Kraft der Brunnen und Bäder.* Aarau, Stuttgart: AT Verlag, 1980.

Halffter, [first name not given]. *Die See-Bade-Anstalten zu Zoppot bei Danzig in ihrem gegenwärtigen Zustande.* Danzig: Wedel'sche Hofbuchdruckerei, 1842.

Hau, Michael. "The Holistic Gaze in German Medicine, 1890-1930," *Bulletin of the History of Medicine* 74 (2000): 495-524.

Haupe, W., ed. *Das Kaiserin-Augusta-Bad in Baden-Baden. Denkschrift zur Erinnerung an die Einweihungsfeier vom 28. Juni, 1893.* Baden-Baden: Ernst Kölblin Hofbuchdruckerei, 1893.

Heidenheimer, Arnold J. "Professional Knowledge and State Policy in Comparative Historical Perspective: Law and Medicine in Britain, Germany and the United States." *International Social Science Journal* 1989 41(4): 529-554.

Heiligenthal, F. *Die Anstalt für mechanische Heilgymnastik im Grossherzoglichen Friedrichsbade in Baden- Baden.* Baden-Baden: A. v. Hagen, 1884.

Heiligenthal, Franz. *Geschichte der Stadt Baden und Ihrer Bäder.* Karlsruhe: Braun'sche Hofbuchdruckerei, 1879.

Hein, Dieter and Andreas Schulz, eds. *Bürgerkultur im 19. Jahrhundert. Bildung, Kunst und Lebenswelt.* Munich: C.H. Beck, 1996.

Heischkel, Edith. "Das Wasser als Arznei in der romantischen Medizin." *Sudhoffs Archiv für Geschichte der Medizin und der Naturwissenschaften* 36 (1952).

Heischkel-Artelt, Edith. "Kurort, Patient und Badearzt in ihrem Zusammenwirken, gezeigt an historischen Beispielen." *Zeitschrift für angewandte Bäder- und Klimaheilkunde* 25, no. 4 (1978): 318-325.

Held-Ritt, Ernst von. *Prißnitz auf Gräfenberg oder treue Darstellung seines Heilverfahrens mit kaltem Wasser: ein Handbuch für alle, welche Gräfenberg besuchen, und der Wasserkur dort oder in die Heimath brauchen wollen so wie für jene, welche dort Heilung fanden.* With an introduction on the history of hydrotherapy and a biography of Priessnitz as well as with explanations and comments, edited by Christian Andree. Expanded second edition of the original, Mörschner u. Jasper, Wien, 1837. Würzburg: Berstadtverlag Korn, 1988.

Hembry, Phyllis, Leonard W. Cowie,and Evelyn E. Cowie, *British Spas from 1815 to the Present: A Social History.* Madison, NJ: Farleigh Dickenson University Press, 1997.

Hembry, Phyllis. *The English Spa 1560-1815: A Social History.* London: Athlone Press, 1990.

Hennemann, H. *Das Sündenregister der Medicinheilkunde.* 2nd expanded edition. St. Gallen: Verlag von Altwegg-Weber zur Treuburg, 1875.

Herwig, Malte. "Magic Science on the Mountain: Science and Myth in Thomas Mann's *Der Zauberberg. Germanic Review* 74, no. 2 (Spring, 1999): 146-156.

Hesse, Hermann. *Kurgast. Aufzeichnungen von einer Badener Kur.* Frankfurt: Suhrkamp Taschenbuchverlag, 1977.

Heyde, Gehard. *Das württembergisch Wunderbad zu Boll; ein geschichtlicher Rückblick nach alten und neuen Quellen.* Stuttgart: J.F. Steinkopf, 1937.

Heyfelder, D. *Die Heilquellen des Grossherzogthums Baden, des Elsaß und des Wasgau.* 1841.

Hirsch, E. *Wie soll der Kranke im Kurorte leben? Ärztliche Ratschläge.* Berlin: Alfred Pulvermacher & Co., medizin. Verlag, 1909.

Hirsch, Emanuel. *Wie soll der Kranke im Kurorte Leben. Ärztliche Ratschläge.* Berlin: Alfred Pulvermacher & Co. medizin. Verlag, 1909.

Hoffmann, Heinrich. *Das Badeort Salzloch* (1860). Project Gutenberg Edition, available at http://gutenberg.spiegel.de/hoffmanh /salzloch/Druckversion_salzloch.htm, accessed on June 19, 2003.

Holborn, Hajo. *A History of Modern Germany, 1840-1945.* Princeton, NJ: Princeton University Press, Paperback Edition, 1982.

Hornekova, Jana. "Karlovarske Kolonady" [The colonnades of Karlovy Vary]. *Umeni a Remesla* [Czechoslavakia] 1975 (1): 24-32.

Houwald, Ernst von. *Vermischte Schriften.* Leipzig: Georg Joachim Göschen, 1825.

Hudemann-Simon, Calixte. *Die Eroberung der Gesundheit, 1750-1900,* trans. from French into German by Andrea van Dülmen. Frankfurt: Fischer, 2000.

Huerkamp, Claudia. "Ärzte und Patienten" in Alfons Labisch and Reinhard Spree, eds., *Medizinische Deutungsmacht im sozialen Wandel des 19. und 20. Jahrhunderts.* Bonn: Psychiatrie Verlag, 1989.

—. "Ärzte und Professionalisierung in Deutschland. Überlegungen zum Wandel des Arztberufs im 19. Jahrhundert." in *Geschichte und Gesellschaft* 6, no. 1 (1980)

—. *Der Aufstieg der Ärzte 19. Jahrhundert.* Göttingen, Vanderhoeck & Ruprecht, 1985.

—. "Die preußisch-deutsche Ärzteschaft als Teil des Bildungsbürgertums." In Werner Conze and Jürgen Kocka, eds., *Bildungsbürgertum im 19. Jahrhundert, Teil 1, Bildungssystem und Professionalisierung im internationalen Vergleichen.* Stuttgart: Klett-Cotta, 1985.

—. "Die preußisch-deutsche Ärzteschaft als Teil des Bildungsbürgertums." In: Werner Conze and Jürgen Kocka, eds. *Bildungsbürgertum im 19. Jahrhundert,* Vol. 1. Stuttgart: Klett-Cotta, 1985, 358-387.

—. "The Making of the Medical Profession, 1800-1914: Prussian doctors in the 19th Century." in Geoffrey Cocks and Konrad Jarausch (eds) *German Professions* Oxford, 1990: 66-84.

—. "Medizinische Lebensreform im späten 19. Jahrhundert: die Naturheilbewegung in Deutschland als Protest gegen die naturwissenschaftliche Universitätsmedizin." *Vierteljahrschrift fur Sozial- und Wirtschaftsgeschichte* 1986 73(2): 158-182.

Hüfner, Gerhard. *Die wissenschaftlichen Vereinigungen im deutschen Heilbäderwesen 1878-1994.* Gütersloh: Flottmann Verlag, 1994.

Jacob, Wolfgang. "Virchows Begriff der 'naturwissenschaftlichen Methode'–Deutung und Grenzen" in *Wege der Naturforschung 1822-1970 im Spiegel der Versammlungen Deutscher Naturforscher und Ärzte*, Hans Querner and Heinrich Schipperges, eds. Berlin, Heidelberg: Springer Verlag, 1972.

Jessen, Jens. *Bibliographie der Selbstzeugnisse deutscher Mediziner, Erinnerungen, Tagebücher und Briefe.* Munich: Saur, 1986.

Jones, Colin. "The Great Chain of Buying: Medical Advertisement, the Bourgeois Public Sphere and the Origins of the French Revolution." *The American Historical Review* 101, no. 1 (February, 1996): 13-40.

Jordan, Herbert. *Udluft-Schemata: Beilage zum Baderbuch der Deutschen Demokratischen Republik.* Leipzig: G. Thieme, 1967.

Jungs, Johann Heinrich [Jung-Stilling]. *Lebensgeschichte oder dessen Jugend, Jünglingsjahre, Wanderschaft, Lehrjahre, häusliches Leben und Alter. Eine wahrhafte Geschichte von ihm selbst erzählt.* Edited and with an introduction bz Max Mendheim. Leipzig: Philipp Reclam jun., [year?]

Jütte, Robert. *Geschichte der alternativen Medizin. Von der Volksmedizin zu den unkonventionellen Therapien von heute.* Munich, C.H. Beck, 1996.

Kaschuba, Wolfgang. "Deutsche Bürgerlichkeit nach 1800. Kultur als symbolische Praxis." In Jürgen Kocka, ed., *Bürgertum im 19. Jahrhundert. Band II: Wirtschaftsbürger und Bildungsbürger.* Göttingen: Vandenhock & Ruprecht, 1995.

Kater, Michael H. "Hitler's Early Doctors: Nazi Physicians in Predepression Germany," *Journal of Modern History* 59, no. 1 (March 1987).

—. "Professionalization and Socialization of Physicians in Wilhelmine and Weimar Germany." *Journal of Contemporary History,* 20, no. 4 (October, 1985).

—. *Doctors under Hitler.* Chapel Hill: University of North Carolina Press, 1989.

Kessel, Martina. "The 'Whole Man:' The Longing for a Masculine World in Nineteenth-Century Germany," *Gender & History* 15, no. 1 (April, 2003): 1-31.

—. *Langeweile. Zum Umgang mit Zeit und Gefühlen in Deutschland vom späten 18. bis zum frühen 20. Jahrhundert.* Göttingen: Wallstein, 2001.

Klein, Christian. *Das Bden. Ein Wort an Gesunde und Kranke.* 2nd edition. Düsseldorf: C. Schaffnit, 1895.

Kleinhempel, Friedrich. *Bäder, Barbiere, Friseure : Geschichte und Geschichten aus uraltem Handwerk.* Frankfurt/Main : R.G. Fischer, 1996.

Kloucek, Viktoria. *Hydro-, Balneo- und Klimatotherapie im Spiegel der Münchner Medizinischen Wochenschrift von 1886- 1900.* Unpublished dissertation. Munich, 1985.

Klüber, Johann Ludwig. *Baden bei Rastatt, nach den unterirdischen Gängen und Kammern des Schlosses, nach den neuesten und künftigen, und nach den ehemaligen römischen öffentlichen Gebäuden und Anlagen der Stadt.* Tübingen: Cotta'sche Buchhandlung, 1807.

Koch, Eduard Josef. *Die Mineral-Quellen Deutschlands und der Schweiz, nebst einem Anhange über die deutschen Nord- und Ostseebäder, naturhistorisch und ärztlich dargestellt.* Vienna: Braumüller & Siedel, 1844.

Kocka, Jürgen. "The Middle Classes in Europe." *The Journal of Modern History* 67, no. 4 (December, 1995): 783-806.

—. *Das lange 19. Jahrhundert. Arbeit, National und bürgerliche Gesellschaft.* Tenth Edition. Gebhard Handbuch der deutschen Geschichte, vol. 13, Rolf Häfele, editor. Stuttgart: Klett-Cotta, 2004.

Kölreuter, W.L., ed. *Die Mineralquellen im Großherzogthum Baden, deren Heilkräfte und Heilanstalten.* 1820.

Kölreuter, Wilhelm Ludwig. *Die Mineralquellen im Großherzogthum Baden, deren Heilkräfte und Heilanstalten in einer Sammlung medizinisch-theoretischer und praktischer Abhandlungen, zur Förderung für Wissenschaft und Kunst in diesem Theile der Heilkunde und zum Leitfaden und Nutzen für Kranke, die an diesen Quellen Hülfe suchen.* Karlsruhe und Baden: D.R. Marx'sche Buchhandlung, 1820.

Konze Werner and Jürgen Kocka, et al. eds., *Bildungbürgertum im 19. Jahrhundert.* 4 volumes. Stuttgart: Klett-Cotta, 1985-92

Kopf, Josef von. *Lebenserinnerungen eines Bildhauers.* Stuttgart and Leipzig: Deutsche Verlagsanstalt, 1899.

Korth, Leonard, ed. *Baden-Baden in der ersten Hälfte des 19. Jahrhunderts.* Baden-Baden: J. Pfeiffer, 1911.

Kragh, Helge. *An Introduction to the Historiography of Science.* Cambridge: Cambridge University Press, 1987.

Kramer, [first name not given]. *Ueber die Eigenschaften, Wirkungen, und den zweckmäßigen Gebrauch der warmen Mineralquelle so wie der natürlichen Stahlbäder zu Baden in Großherzogthume.* Karlsruhe und Baden: Marx'sche Buch- und Kunsthandlung, 1830.

Krell, David Farrell. *Contagion: Sexuality, Disease, and Death in German Idealism and Romanticism.* Bloomington and Indianapolis: Indiana University Press, 1998.

Křížek, Vladímir. *Kulturgeschichte des Heilbades.* Stuttgart and Leipzig: W. Kohlhammer, 1990.

Krüger, Heinrich Eduard. *Dr. Katzenberger's (des Neffen) neue Badereise.* Supplemente zu Jean Paul, vol. 2. Leipzig: E. Wengler, 1858.

Kühl, Stefan. *The Nazi Connection: Eugenics, American Racism, and German National Socialism.* New York: Oxford University Press, 1994.

Kuhnert, Reinhold P. "Badereisen im 18. Jahrhundert–Sozialleben zur Zeit der Aufklärung," *Journal für Geschichte*, no. 1 (1987): 14-23.

—. *Urbanität auf dem Lande. Badereisen nach Pyrmont im 18. Jahrhundert.* Veröffentlichungen des Max-Planck-Instituts für Geschichte, 77. Göttingen, Vandenhoeck & Ruprecht, 1984.

Labich, Alfons. "Medizin und Soziale Kontrolle: zum Verhältnis von Sozialgeschichte und Soziologie der Medizin am Beispiel neuerer Literatur aus der Bundesrepublik Deutschland mit einem Exkurs: neuere Forschungen zur Medizin im Nationalsozialismus." *Dynamis* [Spain] 1987-88 7-8: 427-459.

Labisch, Alfons and Reinhard Spree, eds. *Medizinische Deutungsmacht im sozialen Wandel des 19. und 20. Jahrhunderts.* Bonn: Psychiatrie Verlag, 1989.

Labisch, Alfons and Spree, Reinhard. "Gesundheitspolitik im 19. und im frühen 20. Jahrhundert –Deutschland und England als Beispiele." *Berichte zur Wissenschaftsgeschichte* 1988 11(1): 45-52.

—. "Neuere Entwicklungen und aktuelle Trends in der Sozialgeschichte der Medizin in Deutschland: Rückschau und Ausblick." *Vierteljahrschrift fur Sozial- und Wirtschaftsgeschichte.* 1997 84(2): 171-210, (3): 305-321.

—. "Sozialgeschichte des allgemeinen Krankenhauses in Deutschland (19. und frühes 20. Jahrhundert). *Historia Hospitalium* 1993-94 19: 287-300.

Labisch, Alfons. "Doctors, Workers and the Scientific Cosmology of the Industrial World: The Social Construction of 'Health' and the 'Homo Hygienicus," *Journal of Contemporary History* 20 (1985), 599-615

Labisch, Alfons. Geschichte, Sozialgeschichte und Soziologie der Medizin: ein imaginäres Streitgespräch mit Christian Probst." *Sudhoffs Archiv* 1996 80(1): 1-27.

Lachmund, Jens and Gunnar Stolberg. *Patientenwelten. Krankheit und Medizin vom späten 18. bis zum frühen 20. Jahrhundert im Spiegel von Autobiographien.* Opladen: Leske & Budrich, 1995.

Laube, Heinrich. "Baden." In *Heinrich Laube, Reise durch das Biedermeier*. Franz Heinrich Körber, ed. Hamburg: Hoffmann und Campe, 1965.

—. "Karlsbad." In *Heinrich Laube, Reise durch das Biedermeier*. Franz Heinrich Körber, ed. Hamburg: Hoffmann und Campe, 1965.

Laun, Friedrich (pseud.) [Friedrich August Schulze], *Glitts Erzählungsabende im ** Bade* (Leipzig, 1821.

Lewald, August. "Bilder aus Baden-Baden" *Morgenblatt für gebildete Leser*, October 12, 1847.

Lifton, Robert Jay. *The Nazi Doctors: Medical Killing and the Psychology of Genocide.* London: Macmillan, 1986.

Lindemann, Mary. *Health and Healing in Eighteenth-Century Germany.* Baltimore: Johns Hopkins U. Pr., 1996. 506 pp.

Loeser, Johann. *Geschichte der Stadt Baden* (Baden-Baden: Sommermeyer, 1891

Loetz, Francisca, *Vom Kraken zum Patienten: "Medikalisierung" und medizinische Vergesellschaftlichung am Beispiel Badens, 1750-1850.* Stuttgart: Steiner, 1993.

Lohff, Brigitte. "Die französische Revolution im Spiegelbild: die Reaktion der deutschen Ärzte auf die Revolution und das Revolutionieren." *Berichte zur Wissenschaftsgeschichte* 1989 12(4): 219-228.

Löwenstein, Adolf. *Humor in der Medicin. Medicinisch-humoristische Vorträge, Gedichte, Räthsel, Epigramme etc.* Berlin: Elwin Staude, 1875.

Lozowski, Adolf. *Die Geschichte von Bad Lippspringe vom Tuberkulose-Kurort zum Allergie-Heilbad : eine literarisch-medizinhistorische Studie*. Ph.D. Dissesrtation, Universität Düsseldorf, 1992.

Mackaman, Douglas P. *Leisure Settings: Bourgeois Culture, Medicine, and the Spa in Modern France*. Chicago: University of Chicago Press, 1998.

—. *Doctoring on Vacation: Medicine and Culture at the Spas of Nineteenth-Century France*. Ph.D. Dissertation, University of California, Berkeley, 1993.

Mączak, Antoni and Hans Jürgen Teuteberg, eds. *Reiseberichte als Quellen europäischer Kulturgeschichte. Aufgaben und Möglichkeiten der historischen Reiseforschung*. Wolfenbütteler Forschungen, vol. 21. Wolfenbüttel: Herzog August Bibliothek, 1982.

Maentel, Thorsten. "Zwischen weltbürgerlicher Aufklärung und stadtbürgerlicher Emanzipation." in Dieter Hein and Andreas Schultz, eds., *Bürgerkultur im 19. Jahrhundert*. Munich: C.H. Beck, 1996.

Mahling, Christoph-Helmut. "Residenzen des Glücks.' Konzert-Unterhaltung-Theater–Unterhaltung in Kurorten des 19. und frühen 20. Jahrhunderts," in Michael Mattheus, ed. *Badeorte und Bäderreisen in Antike, Mittelalter und Neuzeit*. Stuttgart: Steiner, 2001, 81-100.

Mangin, Nathalie. Les Relations Franco-Allemandes et les Bains Mondains d'Outre-Rhin." [Franco-German relations and the watering places of Germany]. *Histoire, Economie et Societe* 1994 13(4): 649-675.

Mann, Heinrich. *Doctor Biebers Versuchung*. in *Gesammelte Werke*, Sigrid Anger, Volker Riedel, eds. Berlin und Weimar: Aufbau-Verlag, 1978, 16: 453-505.

Mann, Thomas. "Einführung in den Zauberberg für Studenten der Universität Princeton," in Thomas Mann, *Der Zauberberg*. Berlin: Deutsche Buch-Gemeinschaft, 1967.

—. *Der Zauberberg*. Berlin: Deutsche Buch-Gemeinschaft, 1967.

Manuel Frey. *Der reinliche Bürger*. Kritische Studien zur Geschichtswissenschaft vol. 119, Helmut Berding, Jürgen Kocka, Hans-Peter Ullmann, Hans-Ulrich Wehler, eds. Göttingen: Vanderhoeck & Ruprecht, 1996.

Marcard, H.M. *Beschreibung von Pyrmont 1-2 und Ergänzungsband mit Kupferstichen*. Leipzig, 1784/85, cited in Kuhnert, "Badereisen im 18. Jahrhundert," 18.

Marcuse, Julian. *Bäder und Badewesen in Vergangenheit und Gegenwart*. 1903.

Marfany, Joan-Luis; Burke, Peter (commentary). "The Invention of Leisure in Early Modern Europe." *Past & Present* [Great Britain] 1997 (156): 174-191.

Martin, Peter. *Salon Europas: Baden-Baden im 19. Jahrhundert.* Konstanz: F. Stadler, 1983.

Masten, Viktoria Louise. *Taking the Waters: Elite Women in English Spa Towns, 1700-1800.* M.A. Thesis, California State University, Long Beach, 1993.

Matheus, Michael, ed. *Badeorte und Bäderreisen in Antike, Mittelalter und Neuzeit.* Mainzer Vorträge 5. Stuttgart: Institut für Geschichtliche Landeskunde and der Universität Mainz/Fritz Steiner Verlag, 2001.

Mathias, Peter. "Time for Work, Time for Play: Relations between Work and Leisure in the Early Modern Period." *Vierteljahrschrift fur Sozial- und Wirtschaftsgeschichte* 1994 81(3): 305-323.

Mattäus, Johann. *de Thermis Marchio-Badensibus.* Strassburg, 1618, excerpted with some linguistic modernization from a 1625 copy in Heiligenthal, *Geschichte der Stadt Baden und Ihrer Bäder*, 51-55.

Mattheus, Michael ed. *Badeorte und Bäderreisen in Antike, Mittelalter und Neuzeit.* Stuttgart: Steiner, 2001.

Maurer, Michael. *Die Biographie des Bürgers. Lebensformen und Denkweisen in der formativen Phase des deutschen Bürgertums (1680-1815).* Veröffentlichungen des Max-Planck-Instituts für Geschichte, 127. Göttingen: Vandenhoeck & Ruprecht, 1996.

McClelland, Charles E. "Modern German Doctors: A Failure of Professionalization?" In Manfred Berg and Geoffrey Cocks, eds., *Medicine and Modernity: Public Health and Medical Care in Nineteenth- and Twentieth-Century Germany.* Washington, DC: German Historical Institute and Cambridge University Press, 1996.

McClelland, Charles E. "Zur Professionalisierung der akademischen Berufe in Deutschland," in *Bildungsbürgertum im 19. Jahrhundert*, ed. Werner Conze and Jürgen Kocka, 233-247. Industrielle Welt. Schriftenreihe des Arbeitskreises für moderne Sozialgeschichte, ed. Werner Conze, No. 38.

—. *The German Experience of Professionalization. Modern Learned Professions and their Organizations from the Early Nineteenth Century to the Hitler Era.* Cambridge, Cambridge University Press, 1991.

Mende, Ludwig Julius Kaspar. "Ueber den Besuch der Bäder und den Nutzen der Mineralwasser" *Monatsschrift für Deutsche* 2 (1801). Accessed electronically from the University of Bielefeld electronic collections on December 20, 2002 at www.ub.uni-bielefeld.de/digibib.aufkl.html.

Mendelssohn, Peter de. *Der Zauberer: Das Leben des deutschen Schriftstellers Thomas Mann*. Frankfurt am Main: Fischer, 1996.

Mettenheim, H. von. "Vom Denken und Handeln der Badeärzte in den Jahren 1850-1898 nach Briefen." *Zeitschrift für angewandte Bäder- und Klimaheilkunde*, 25 (1978): 318-325.

Mikoletzky, Juliane. Zur Sozialgeschichte des Österreichischen Kurorts im 19. Jahrhundert: Kurlisten und Kurtaxordnungen als historische Quelle." *Mitteilungen des Instituts fur Österreichische Geschichtsforschung*. 1991 99(3-4): 393-433.

Mitscherlich, Alexander and Fred Mielke, *Doctors of Infamy; the Story of the Nazi Medical Crimes*. New York: Henry Schuman, 1949.

Moerchel, Joachim. *Die Nassauischen Badeärzte in ihrer wissenschaftlichen und praktischen Tätigkeit 1816-1866*. European University Papers Series VII, Health Sciences-Division B History of Medicine, Vol. 1. Frankfurt am Main: Peter Lang, 1977.

Mohl, Robert von. *Kissingen vor 60 Jahren. Badebriefe eines deutschen Professors. Mit Anmerkungen herausgegeben von Dr. Kerler*. Bad-Kissingen: Friedrich Weinberger, 1903.

Moran, Daniel. *Toward the Century of Words : Johann Cotta and the Politics of the Public Realm in Germany, 1795-1832*. Berkeley: University of California Press, 1990.

—. *Toward the Century of Words : Johann Cotta and the Politics of the Public Realm in Germany, 1795-1832*. Berkeley: University of California Press, 1990.

Mörgeli, Christoph, ed. *Europas Medizin im Biedermeier anhand der Reiseberichte des Züricher Arztes Conrad Meyer-Hofmeister 1827-1831*. Basel: Schwalbe, 1997.

Morin, Friedrich. *Die vorzüglichsten Bäder und Heilquellen Deutschlands und der Nachbarstaaten, deren ärztlichen Hülfen, Einrichtungen, Sehenswürdigkeiten, Vergnügungen und Umgebungen. Ein Rathgeber für Bade-Reisende*. Berlin: Nicolaische Verlagsbuchhandlung, 1867.

Müller-Hill, Benno. *Murderous Science: Elimination by Scientific Selection of Jews, Gypsies, and Others, Germany 1933-1945*. Oxford: Oxford University Press, 1988.

Nicosia, Francis R. and Jonathan Huener, eds. *Medicine and Medical Ethics in Nazi Germany: Origins, Practices, Legacies*. New York: Berghahn Books, 2002.

Niendorf, Emma. [Emma von Suckow], "Villeggiatur in Baden." *Morgenblatt für gebildete Leser,* April 28 1845, 402-403.

Nipperdey, Thomas. *Deutsche Geschichte* 3 volumes, Brochierte Sonderausgabe. Munich: C.H. Beck, 1998.

Nürnberger, Helmuth. *Fontanes Welt*. Berlin: Siedler, 1997.

Nye, Robert A. "The Evolution of the Concept of Medicalization in the Late Twentieth Century." *Journal of History of the Behavioral Sciences* vol. 39, no. 2 (Spring, 2003), 115-129.

Oberschwabische Bader: Bad Buchau, Bad Schussenried, Bad Waldsee, Bad Wurzach, Aulendorf. Berlin: RV Verlag, 1994.

Obkircher, Arnold. *Baden-Baden. Die Thermen und die Grossherzoglichen Kuranstalten.* Karlsruhe: Verlag der Chr. F. Müller'schen Hofbuchhandlung, 1897.

Oefflinger, H. *Die Kurorte und Heilquellen des Grossherzogtums Baden für Aerzte und Heilbedürftige.* Baden-Baden, Sommermeyer, 1905.

Oertel, Eucharius Ferdinand Christian. *Vincenz Priessnitz oder ein Aufruf an alle Staatsregierungen Deutschlands zur Einrichtung von Wasserheilanstalten*. 1834, cited in Prignitz, *Wasserkur und Badelust.*

Ostseebad Zoppot. Führer für Kurgäste. Herausgegeben im Auftrage und unter Mitwirkung der Bade-Direction. Danzig, Verlag von H.L. Alexander's Buchdruckerei, 1886.

Pecht, Friedrich. *Aus Meiner Zeit. Lebenserinnerungen*. Munich: Verlagsanstalt für Kunst und Wissenschaft, 1894.

Peez, A.H. *Ueber den Werth Wiesbadens und einiger andrer Curorte Deutschlands in Bezug auf Winter-Curen und als Winteraufenthalt für Kranke und Schwächliche*. Wiesbaden: J.F. Hassloch'sche Buchhandlung, 1840.

Peters, Hermann. *Der Arzt und die Heilkunst in der deutschen Vergangenheit.* Monographien zur deutschen Kulturgeschichte, Vol. 3, edited by Georg Steinhaufen. Leipzig: Eugen Diderichs, 1900.

Pfeiffer, E. *Wiesbaden als Curort.* 1887.

Porter, Roy, ed. *The Medical History of Waters and Spas.* London: Wellcome Institute for the History of Medicine, 1990.

Pretzel, Ulrike. *Die Literaturform Reiseführer im 19. und 20. Jarhundert. Untersuchungen am Beispiel des Rheins.* Frankfurt/M.: Peter Lang, 1995.

Prignitz, Horst. *Wasserkur und Badelust: Eine Badereise in die Vergangenheit.* Leipzig: Koehler & Amelang, 1986.

Proctor, Robert. *Racial Hygiene: Medicine under the Nazis.* Cambridge, MA: Harvard University Press, 1988.

Püttner, Elise. *Nordostdeutsche Städte und Landschaften, No. 1: Ostseebad Zoppot bei Danzig.* Danzig: A.W. Kafemann, 1887.

Querner, Hans and Heinrich Schipperges, eds. *Wege der Naturforschung 1822-1972 im Spiegel der Versammlungen Deutscher Naturforscher und Ärzte.* Berlin, Heidelberg, New York: Springer Verlag, 1972.

Radkau, Joachim. *Das Zeitalter der Nervösität. Deutschland zwischen Bismarck und Hitler.* Munich: Propyläen, 2000.

Rampold, [no first name given]. *Ueber die Bäder und Kurorte des Königreichs Württemberg.* Reprints from the *Jahrbuücher für Deutschlands Heilquellen und Seebäder,* 1838. Berlin: List und Klemann, 1838.

Regin, Cornelia. "Zwischen Angriff und Abwehr. Die Naturheilbewegung als medizinkritische Öffentlichkeit im Deutschen Kaiserreich." in Martin Dinges, ed., *Medizinkritische Bewegungen im Deutschen Reich (ca. 1870–ca. 1933).* MedGG Beihefte 9. Stuttgart: Steiner Verlag, 1996.

Reimann, Helga. "The Informal Code: Changes in Western Etiquette." *Thought* 1989 64(252): 41-50.

Reise-Handbuch für die christliche Familie. Ein Wegweiser durch Hospize, Erholungshäuser, Pensionen, Hotels, Sanatorien, Sommerfrischen, Bäder, Kurorte, nebst praktischen Auskünften für die Reise, Seventeenth Edition. Berlin: Vaterländische Verlags- und Kunstanstalt, 1912.

Richter, Gustav Heinrich. *Kur- und Lebensregeln für Wiesbaden's Brunnengäste.* Düsseldorf: J.H.C. Schreiner, 1842.

—. *Wiesbaden als heilsamer Aufenthaltsort für Schwache und Kranke aus dem Norden Europa's und als Kurort für jede Jahreszeit mit besonderer Bezugnahme auf die Zuslässigkeit des Gebrauchs von Winterkuren.* Elberfeld: Schönian'sche Buchhandlung, 1839.

Richter, Jean Paul Friedrich (Jean Paul), *Auswahl aus des Teufels Papieren*. In *Jean Paul's sämmtliche Werke,* 1828.

—. (Jean Paul), *Dr. Katzenbergers Badereise*, in *Jean Paul's sämmtliche Werke*, LI, vol. 1-3. Berlin: Reimer, 1828.

Ridder, Paul. *Im Spiegel der Arznei: Sozialgeschichte der Medizin* Stuttgart: S. Hirzel, 1990. 287 pp.

Ringer, Fritz K. *The Decline of the German Mandarins: The German Academic Community, 1890-1933.* Cambridge, MA: Harvard University Press, 1969.

Risse, Günter B. "Philosophical' Medicine in Nineteenth-Century Germany: An Episode in the Relations between Philosophy and Medicine." *Journal of Medicine and Philosophy* 1, no. 1 (1976).

Rohde, J. "In Vergessenheit geratene Erkenntnisse über Priessnitz aus dem unbekannt gebliebenen Vinzenz Priessnitz'schen Familien-Wasserbuch von 1847," *Forschende Komplementärmedizin und Klassische Naturheilkunde* 9 (2002).

Rössler, Oskar. *Baden-Baden als Heilbad. Gesammelte Aufsätze.* Baden-Baden: Ernst Brockhoff, 1936

Rudolph, Gerhard. "100 Jahre wissenschaftliche Balneologie." Keynote Lecture at the 83rd Congress of the Deutsche Gesellschaft für Physikalische Medizin und Rehabilitation, October 13, 1978 in Berlin, reproduced in Gerhard Rudolph, *Zwei Beiträge zur Geschichte der Balneologie.* Kassel: Verlag Hans Meister KG, 1982.

—. *Zwei Beiträge zur Geschichte der Balneologie. Die kulturgeschichtlichen und medizinischen Wurzeln des Bäderwesens. 100 Jahre wissenschaftliche Balneologie.* Kassel: Verlag Hans Meister, 1982.

Ruef, A. *Das Lithium und die lithiumhaltigen Quellen von Baden-Baden als wirksames Heilmittel gegen Gicht.* Baden-Baden: Hofbuchhandlung von J.R. Marx, 1862.

Rullmann, G.C.W. *Wiesbaden und seine Heilquellen für Curgäste beschrieben.* Wiesbaden: Ludwig Schellenberg, Hofbuchhändler und Hofbuchdrucker, 1823.

Schadewaldt, H. "Das Badewesen in der Goethezeit." *Therapiewoche* 32 (1982): 4123-4133.

Schallmayer, Egon. *Aquae, das römische Baden-Baden.* Stuttgart: K. Theiss, 1989.

Schipperges, Heinrich. "Repräsentative Eröffnungsreden auf den Naturforscherversammlungen im 19. Jahrhundert" in *Wege der Naturforschung*, 12.

—. *Utopien der Medizin. Geschichte und Kritik der ärztlichen Ideologie des 19. Jahrhunderts.* Salzburg, Otto Müller Verlag, 1968.

Schlich, Thomas. 'Medicalization and Secularization: the Jewish Ritual Bath as a Problem of Hygiene (Germany, 1820s - 1840s). *Social History of Medicine* 1995 8(3): 423-442.

Schmitter, Annette. *Die Anfänge der Entwicklung einer naturwissenschaftlichen Begründung der Balneologie am Beispiel des Wirkens Friedrich Wilhelm Benekes als Badearzt in (Bad) Nauheim.* M.D. dissertation, Rheinisch-Westfälische Technische Hochschule Aachen, 1986.

Schmuhl, Hans-Walter. *Rassenhygiene, Nationalsozialismus, Euthanasie: von der Verhütung zur Vernichtung "lebensunwerten Lebens," 1890-1945.* Göttingen: Vanderhoeck & Ruprecht, 1987.

Schnitzler, Arthur. *Doktor Gräsler, Badearzt.* Frankfurt am Main: Fischer, 1997.

Schreiber, Alois. *Le Guide du Voyage du Rhin*, L'Abbé Henry trans. Nouvelle Edition Considérablement Augmentée. Heidelberg, 1818.

—. *Le Guide du Voyage du Rhin, Nouvelle Edition Considérablement Augmentée.* L'Abbé Henry trans. [Original title: *Handbuch für Reisende am Rhein*]Heidelberg, 1818.

Schreiber, H. *Handbuch für Eisenbahn-Reisende durch das Grossherzogthum Baden, nebst den Reiserouten durch das Neckarthal, über den Schwarzwald und nach den Seegegenden.* Karlsruhe, Chr. Fr. Müller'sche Hofbuchhandlung, 1846.

Schreiber, Hippolyt. *Aurelia. Bilder und Träume aus Baden und der Umgegend.* Baden, 1844.

Shorter, Edward. "Private Clinics in Central Europe, 1850-1933," *Social History of Medicine* 3, no. 2 (1990): 159-195.

Sievert, Lars Endrik. *Naturheilkunde und Medizinethik im Nationalsocialismus.* Frankfurt am Main: Mabuse-Verlag, 1996.

Simon, J. Franz. *Die Heilquellen Europa's mit vorzüglicher Berücksichtigung ihrer chemischen Zusammensetzung.* Berlin: Albert Förstner, 1839.

—. *Die Heilquellen Europa's mit vorzüglicher Berücksichtigung ihrer chemischen Zusammensetzung nach ihrem physikalischen und medizinischen Verhalten.* 1839.

Snellman, Joh. *Dt. E. Reise durch die deutschsprachigen Ländern*, vols. 1 & 2, 1840-1841.

Sommer, Hermann . *Zur Kur Nach Ems. Ein Beitrag zur Geschichte der Baderise von 1830 bis 1914.* Geschichtliche Landeskunde, Bd. 48, Franz Steiner Verlag, Stuttgart, 1999.

—. "Stationen eines Kurbads im 19. Jahrhundert–Bad Ems," in Michael Mattheus, ed. *Badeorte und Bäderreisen in Antike, Mittelalter und Neuzeit.* Stuttgart: Steiner, 2001, 101-132.

Spalteholz, R. *Eine Badereise. Lustspiel in 4 Aufzügen.* Leipzig: Oswald Mutze, 1881.

Spengler, L., ed. *Die Verhandlungen der deutschen Gesellschaft für Hydrologie während ihrer ersten Generalversammlung zu Berlin am 1. und 2. Mai 1855.* Wetzlar: Verlag von G. Rathgeber, 1855.

Sponagel, Georg Christian. *Meine viertägigen Leiden im Bade zu Pyrmont. Eine Brunnen-Lektüre.* 3rd unaltered edition. Pyrmont: Georg Uslar, 1824

Sterngass, Jon. *First Resorts: Pursuing Pleasure at Saratoga Springs, Newport, and Coney Island.* Baltimore : Johns Hopkins University Press, 2001.

Steudel, Johannes. "Geschichte der Bäder- und Klimaheilkunde" in Walther Amelung and Arrien Evers, eds. *Handbuch der Bäder- und Klimaheilkunde.* Stuttgart: Schattauer, 1962.

Stollberg, Gunnar. "Die Naturheilvereine im deutschen Kaiserreich." *Archiv für Sozialgeschichte* 1988 28: 287-305.

Storm, Theodor. *Ein Bekenntnis.* Chemnitz: H. Thümmlers Verlag, [1887].

Struck, Wolf-Heino. *Wiesbaden im Biedermeyer.* Wiesbaden, 1981.

Studt, Birgit. "Die Badenfahrt. Ein Neues Muster der Badepraxis und Badegeselligkeit." In: Michael Matheus, ed., *Badeorte und Bäderreisen in Antike, Mittelalter und Neuzeit.* Mainzer Vorträge 5. Stuttgart: Institut für Geschichtliche Landeskunde and der Universität Mainz/Fritz Steiner Verlag, 2001.

Stürzbrecher, Manfred. *Deutsche Ärztebriefe des 19. Jahrhunderts.* Göttingen: Musterschmidt, 1975.

Sul, Heasim. *Commercialization of Leisure: English Spa Towns in the Sixteenth and the Seventeenth Centuries.* Ph.D. Dissertation, University of California, Irvine, 1995

Tamm, Ingo. *Ärzte und gesetzliche Krankenversicherung in Deutschland und England, 1880-1914.* Berlin: Verlag für Wissenschafts- und Regionalgeschichte Dr. Michael Engel, 1988.

Taschenbuch für Badereisende. Jahrbuch der Bäder, Curorte, Heilanstalten 1873, 5. verbesserte Auflage. Berlin: Denicke's Verlag, 1873.

Thilenius, Hartman Christian. *Ems und seine Heilquellen für Bade- und Brunnengäste beschrieben und mit einer Anleitung zu ihren zweckmäßigen Gebrauche versehen.* Wiesbaden: Schellenberg, 1816.

Thomsen, Peter. *Ärzte auf dem Weg ins "Dritte Reich:" Studien zur Arbeitsmarktsituation, zum Selbstverständnis und zur Standespolitik der Ärzteschaft gegenüber der Sozialversicherung während der Weimarer Republik.* Historische Studien, Band 447, Helmut Castitius, Reinhard Elze, Eberhard Jäckel et al., eds. Husum: Matthiesen, 1996.

Titzmann, Oliver. *Radiumbad Oberschlema: die Geschichte eines Kurortes.* Schlema: Kurgesellschaft, 1995.

Toellner, Richard. "Die wissenschaftliche Ausbildung des Arztes is eine Culturfrage...' Über das Verhältnis von Wissenschaftsanspruch, Bildungsprogramme und Praxis der Medizin." *Berichte zur Wissenschaftsgeschichte* 1988 11(4): 193-205.

Toepfer, Karl. *Der reiche Mann, oder: die Wasserkur. Schauspiel in vier Aufzügen.* Berlin: Theater-Buchhandlung Eduard Bloch, 1873.

Travis, John Frederick. *The Rise of Holidaymaking on the Devon Coast, 1750 to 1900, with Particular Reference to Health and Entertainment.* (Vols. I and II). Ph.D. Dissertation, University of Exeter, 1988.

Tsouyopoulos, Nelly. *Andreas Roschlaub und die Romantische Medizin: Die philosophischen Grundlagen der Modernen Medizin*. Stuttgart: Gustav Fischer, 1982. 259 pp.

Tuchman, Arleen Marcia. *Science, Medicine and the State: The Institutionalization of Scientific Medicine at the University of Heidelberg*. Ph.D Dissertation, U. of Wisconsin, Madison 1985.

—. *Science, Medicine and the State in Germany. The Case of Baden, 1815-1871*. New York, Oxford: Oxford University Press, 1993.

Turgenev, Ivan. *Rauch*. Translated from Russian into German by Dieter Pommerenke. Berlin: Aufbau Taschenbuchverlag, 1997.

Tustin, Joseph Philips. *Bad Kissingen: story of a spa*. 1st ed. Germany. Printed by T.A. Schachenmayer Print-Shop, 1947.

Valenza, Janet Mace. *Places Lived, Places Lost: Taking the Waters in Texas*. Ph.D. Dissertation, The University of Texas at Austin, 1992.

Varnhagen, Rahel. *Briefwechsel.* 4 vols. Edited by Friedhelm Kemp. Munich: Winkler Verlag, 1979.

Virchow, Rudolf. *Sämtliche Werke*, Christian Andree, ed. Band 59, Abteilung IV: Briefwechsel mit den Eltern 1839-1864, zum ersten Mal vollständig in historisch-kritischer Edition. Berlin, Vienna: Blackwell Wissenschafts-Verlag, 2001.

Vollmer, Emil. *Meine Erinnerungen.* Bad Kreuznach: Harrach, 1935.

Waddington, Ivan. "Medicine, the market and professional autonomy: some aspects of the professionalization of medicine," in *Bildungsbürgertum im 19. Jahrhundert*, ed. Werner Conze and Jürgen Kocka, 388-416. Industrielle Welt. Schriftenreihe des Arbeitskreises für moderne Sozialgeschichte, ed. Werner Conze, No. 38.

Waetzel, Paul, ed. *Baden-Baden: Neuester Führer durch die Stadt und Ihre Umgegend.* Baden-Baden: Friedrich Spies, 1898.

Walton, John and Smith, Jenny. "The First Spanish Seaside Resorts." *History Today* 1994 44(8): 23-29.

Wandrey, Horst, ed. *Die Frau des Arztes. Erzählungen um Arztschicksale aus zwei Jahrhunderten.* Berlin: Buchverlag der Morgen, 1964.

Weber, Eugen. "Introduction: Decadence on a a Private Income." *Journal of Contemporary History* 1982 17(1): 1-20 .

Wehler, Hans-Ulrich. *Deutsche Gesellschaftsgeschichte, Dritter Band: Von der "Deutschen Doppelrevolution bis zum Beginn des Ersten Weltkrieges, 1849-1914.* Munich: C.H. Beck, 1995.

Weindling, Paul. "Bourgeois values, doctors and the state: the professionalization of medicine in Germany, 1848-1933." In David Blackbourn and Richard J. Evans, eds., *The German Bourgeoisie.*

Essays on the German middle class from the late eighteenth to the early twentieth century. London and New York: Routledge, 1991.

—. “Medicine and Modernization: The Social History of German Health and Medicine.” *History of Science* 24 (1986) 277-301.

—. *Health, Race, and German Politics between National Unification and Nazism, 1870-1945*. Cambridge, New York: Cambridge University Press, 1989.

—. “Shattered Alternatives in Medicine.” *History Workshop Journal* 1983 (16): 152-157.

Weis, Johann Baptist. *Hans-Jörgels Badereise*, Vols. 1 & 2. Vienna: Bauer und Dirnböck, 1842.

Weller, K. *Taschenbuch für Badereisende. Jahrbuch der Bäder, Curorte, Heilanstalten 1873*. 5. verbesserte Auflage. Berlin: Denicke’s Verlag, 1873.

Welper, [no first name given]. *Die wichtigen Bäder Euzropa’s. Zur Empfehlung der Bäder für Gesunde und Kranke*. Berlin, 1820.

Wetzler, Johann Evangelist. *Über Gesundbrunnen und Heilbäder*. Mainz, 1825.

Widmann, Martin. *Bäder und Wundarzt : medizinhistorisches Handwerk in vergangenen Tagen*. Zürich: Medizinhistorisches Institut der Universität Zürich, 1998.

Wie soll der gesunde und kranke Kurgast im Ostseebade leben? Ein Wegweiser für die Badegäste der Ostsee. Berlin, 1905.

Wiesbaden als heilsamer Aufenthaltsort für Schwache und Kranke ...Elberfeld, 1839.

Wieser, Walter G. “Das Literarische Baden.” [The literary Baden]. *Biblos* [Austria] 1977 26(2): 157-163.

Wiesing, Urban. Die Einsamkeit des Arztes un der ‘lebendige Drang nach Geschichte’: zum historischen Selbstverständis der Medizin bei Richard Koch.” *Gesnerus* 1997 54(3-4): 219-241.

Wisbaden Recommended to the Gouty and Rheumatic, by a Fellow-Sufferer. London: James Ridgeway and Sons, Piccadilly, 1837.

Wolfschmidt, Gudrun, ed. *Popularisierung der Naturwissenschaften*. Berlin: Verlag für Geschichte der Naturwissenschaften und der Technik, 2002.

Woycke, James. “Patent Medicines in Imperial Germany.” *Canadian Bulletin of Medical History* 1992 9(1): 41-56.

Yegül, Fikret K. “The Thermo-Mineral Complex at Baiae and De Balneis Puteolanis,” *Art Bulletin*, 78, no. 1 (March 1996).

Ziegler, Uwe. "Die württembergischen Badeorte im 19. Jahrhundert." *Zeitschrift für Württembergische Landesgeschichte* 41 (1982): 201-214.

Ziolkowski, Theodore. *German Romanticism and Its Institutions.* Princeton: Princeton University Press, 1990.

Zipperlen, Johann Bernhard. *Hülfsbüchlein für Gesundheitslehre für alle Stände. Eine gemeinnützige Anleitung zum wirksamen Gebrauch des kalten Wassers.* Stuttgart: Verlag der J.F. Steintopf'schen Buchhandlung, 1844.

Zwierlein, K.A. *Ueber die neuesten Badeanstalten in Deutschland.* 1843.

INDEX

allopathic medicine 2, 11, 119, 120, 131, 142
American spas 74, 148
antisemitism 125, 148-153
Armenbad (Poor Bath) 34-35, 71, 113
Asclepios (Asclepieion) 15, 44
Aurelia Aquensis 14, 15, 23, 27, 44, 45, 103
Austria 5, 13, 61, 73, 78, 96, 140, 163
Baden im Aargau 16, 17
Baden-Baden 3, 5, 6, 7, 12, 13, 14, 16, 17, 22, 23, 25, 27-38, 40-47, 61-71, 82, 88, 90, 93, 95-116, 121, 124-128, 137-140, 143-145, 147-150
Baiae 14-15
balneology 3, 8, 9, 62, 85, 89, 90-93, 96, 106, 108, 110, 119, 122-124, 128-129, 134, 141
baths, bathing 5, 7, 11, 13-17, 22, 23, 25, 26, 28, 30, 34-38, 42, 44, 45, 48, 49, 51, 52, 53, 61, 62, 64, 67, 68, 70-74, 77, 81, 83, 88, 102, 103, 104, 107, 108, 111, 112, 113, 115, 138, 140, 155-156, 161-164
Bebel, Heinrich 17, 39
Bildung 39, 58-59, 109
Bismarck, Otto von 11, 72-74, 77, 84, 91, 99, 119
Blitz, Rudolf 124-127, 128, 129
Brentano, Clemens 40
Bürgertum, bürgerlich - see middle class
businessmen 27, 62, 63, 98, 99, 111, 131, 134,
Caracalla 23
casino and gaming 31-32, 38-39, 49, 52, 65, 66-68, 79, 95-105, 107, 111, 115, 112, 138-140, 147
end of 95-105
charlatans, charlatanism 25, 50, 75, 90, 91, 127, 128, 130
Chèzy, Wilhelm von 63-64, 68
Cicero 14, 16
concerts 31, 33, 42, 106
Cotta, Johann Friedrich 36, 41, 42, 44
Dostoevsky, Fyodor 64, 65, 95 note, 98
drinking cure 17, 19, 21, 26, 34, 46, 48, 49, 52, 71, 76, 79, 83, 158-161
Ems (Bad Ems) 5, 13, 28, 37, 41, 61, 82, 85, 90, 97, 100, 110, 115, 137, 138
exclusivity 12, 18, 21, 31, 39, 113, 114, 115
experimental medicine 45, 85-87, 90, 120, 141
France 5, 13, 27, 62, 96, 111, 125, 127
Frech, Karl 72, 100, 101, 102, 103, 105
Friedrichsbad 102-104, 107, 108, 112, 114, 145
gardens (*Kurgarten*) 18, 19, 30, 32-33, 37, 42, 52, 53, 54
Goethe, Wolfgang von 7, 11, 36, 40, 81, 105
Gräfenberg 78-82
guest registries - see *Kurliste*
guidebooks 6, 22, 34, 41, 44-52, 54, 56, 64, 66, 68-69, 74, 81, 82-83, 84, 90, 105-106, 108-110, 116, 141

Hadrian 23, 103
health insurance 9, 112-114, 119, 144, 146, 152
Heiligenthal, Franz 68, 105, 107, 109
Hoffmann, Heinrich 91-92
homeopathy 118, 119, 142, 144
horse racing 100
hotels 5, 7, 30, 35-36, 40-42, 52, 54, 69-72, 98, 113, 114, 115, 148, 149
Jung-Stilling, Heinrich 40
Kaiserin-Augusta-Bad 112
Karl Friedrich, Grand Duke of Baden 28
Karlsbad (Karlovy Vary) 5, 43, 61, 75, 96, 115, 140, 155, 157, 158
Klüber, Johann Ludwig 36, 42, 44
Kneipp, Sebastian 120-121, 129, 142
Kölreuter, Wilhelm Ludwig 47-49
Kurliste 27, 40, 106
Landesbad (Public Bath) 113-115, 144
landscape 19, 33, 54, 66, 69, 137
Laube, Heinrich 67, 74, 75, 163
lay practitioners 3, 7, 50, 62, 78-82, 93, 120-122, 124, 128, 129, 142, 145
Lewald, August 65-66, 70
Mann, Heinrich 130 ff
Mann, Thomas 131 ff
medical authority 2, 8, 9, 49-51, 54, 56-59, 63, 73, 79, 82, 83, 93, 94, 103, 117, 118, 121, 127, 128, 130, 133, 142-146, 152
medicalization 2, 3, 5, 8, 146
Middle Ages 15, 27, 44
middle-class (also *Bürgertum*, *bürgerlich*) 1, 2, 4, 6, 19, 20, 21, 22, 26, 27, 31, 33, 39-43, 53-54, 57-58, 59, 62, 67, 70, 129, 135, 139, 145
Morgenblatt für gebildete Stände 7, 42-44, 55, 65-66, 73, 96, 100, 139
nationalism 72, 103, 111, 145
neurasthenia 116-118, 130, 145
nobles, nobility 16, 18, 20, 21, 27, 33, 39, 40, 43, 53, 57, 59, 70, 79, 98, 99
notables, visits by 39, 40, 70, 80, 126
pastors 27
Paul, Jean - see Richter, Jean Paul Friedrich
physicians 3-9, 14, 19, 23, 25-27, 29, 32, 35, 37, 41, 43, 45-59, 62, 71-72, 73, 74, 75- 78, 80, 81, 82-85, 87-93, 94, 96, 100, 101-102, 104, 106, 109-110, 115-124, 127-135, 137-147, 150-153
Plombières 13, 96
poor 18, 19, 20, 27, 34-35, 39, 55, 56, 71, 113-115, 126
Priessnitz, Vincenz 3, 78-82, 89, 93, 94, 121-122, 129, 140, 142
private clinics 5, 114, 117, 130-132, 144, 145
professionalization 2-6, 8, 9, 50, 58, 59, 120, 122-124, 128, 132, 140-142, 146
professors 27, 75, 90, 125, 129
Promenadenordnung 32, 39, 54
promotion 12, 18-19, 23, 26, 29, 30, 41-50, 85, 89, 106-111, 137
  medical studies as 18-19, 41, 45-50, 109
prostitution 33, 39, 67
Pyrmont 20, 22, 28, 37, 38
quackery 9, 80, 83, 90, 118, 120, 124, 126, 127, 142, 143
railroads 62, 63, 69, 116, 139. 156
Richter, Gustav Heinrich 71, 82-84
Richter, Jean Paul Friedrich 55-56, 58, 164
Roman Empire 11, 14-15
Roman legacy 15, 22-23, 34, 44, 102-103, 108
Romantic medicine 8, 39, 45-46, 55, 93, 119, 133, 141
Romanticism 22, 110

Röschlaub, Andreas 45
rules of conduct - see
    Promenadenordnung
Rullmann, G.C.W. 38, 48-49, 54, 56
Saratoga Springs 74
Schelling, Friedrich Wilhelm 8, 45, 55, 58, 86 note,
Seneca 13-14
sex and sexuality 16, 33, 44, 54, 118
    licentiousness 14, 16, 67
    and illicit affairs (*Kurschatten*) 67
social interaction 1, 14, 20-22, 26, 33, 38, 40, 52, 53, 72
spa
    doctors (*Badeärzte*) 5, 8, 23, 25, 32, 41, 45, 46, 48, 50, 52, 54, 55, 57-59, 62, 73, 77-79, 81-85, 87-89, 91, 93-94, 101-102, 110, 121-124, 127-129, 133-134, 137 ff, 142, 146, 151, 152
    freedom (*Badefreiheit*) 22, 43, 54, 67, 141
    administration 3, 5-8, 29, 31-36, 38-40, 41, 45-47, 62, 64, 66-67, 69, 70, 88, 86, 104, 106, 124, 128, 137-139, 144
    aristocratic 19-22
    development as a state interest 5, 29
    satire of 55-56, 74-77, 91-92, 155-164
    Conversation House (*Conversationshaus*) 30-34, 37, 42, 48, 52, 53, 64, 65, 98-100, 138, 147
spa definition 13 ff
spa medicine 3, 6, 8, 12, 45-46, 58, 62, 77, 78, 81, 85, 86, 88-91, 93, 94, 121, 122, 127-130, 141
Spengler, Ludwig 90, 122-123
sponsorship, state 18, 22, 28, 37, 139, 140
students 27, 66, 134, 150, 152
Suckow, Emma von (Emma Niendorf) 65, 96
syphilis 17, 67, 84
Tepliz (Cieplice) 61, 140, 158
theater 5, 14, 15, 30, 33, 42, 49, 104
thermae 11, 14, 15, 102, 103
Thilenius, Georg 122-123, 129
Tieck, Ludwig 40
Trinkhalle 21, 30, 34, 38, 44, 52, 53, 56, 72, 74, 138
Turgenev, Ivan 95, 96, 100, 139
Uhland, Ludwig 40
universities, spa medicine and 46, 50, 57-58, 93, 119, 122, 126, 129, 134, 142-143
Varnhagen, Rahel 40, 53, 55-56
vice 15, 38, 65, 67, 68, 93, 95 ff.
Vichy 5, 13, 61, 96
Virchow, Rudolf 72, 74, 86-88, 93, 143
Weinbrenner, Friedrich 29, 31, 33, 34, 36
Wiesbaden 5, 12, 13, 16, 18, 25, 28, 37, 38, 41, 43, 46-49, 54, 59, 61, 63, 64, 70-72, 82-83, 85, 87, 97, 101, 107, 109, 110, 115, 122, 137-140, 149
Zipperlen, Johann Bernhard 81-82
Zoppot (Sopot) 13, 37
Zwierlein, K.A. 25, 26, 48, 78